Becoming a Subject

Becoming a Subject

Reflections in Philosophy and Psychoanalysis

MARCIA CAVELL

CLARENDON PRESS · OXFORD

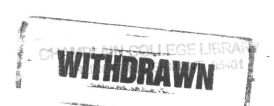

OXFORD
UNIVERSITY PRESS

Great Clarendon Street, Oxford OX2 6DP

Oxford University Press is a department of the University of Oxford.
It furthers the University's objective of excellence in research, scholarship,
and education by publishing worldwide in

Oxford New York

Auckland Cape Town Dar es Salaam Hong Kong Karachi
Kuala Lumpur Madrid Melbourne Mexico City Nairobi
New Delhi Shanghai Taipei Toronto

With offices in

Argentina Austria Brazil Chile Czech Republic France Greece
Guatemala Hungary Italy Japan Poland Portugal Singapore
South Korea Switzerland Thailand Turkey Ukraine Vietnam

Oxford is a registered trade mark of Oxford University Press
in the UK and in certain other countries

Published in the United States
by Oxford University Press Inc., New York

British Library Cataloguing in Publication Data

Data available

Library of Congress Cataloging in Publication Data

Cavell, Marcia, 1931–
Becoming a subject : reflections in philosophy and psychoanalysis / Marcia Cavell.
p. cm.
Includes bibliographical references and index.
1. Psychoanalysis and philosophy. 2. Subjectivity. I. Title.
BF175.4.P45C375 2006 150.19'5—dc22 2005033563

Typeset by Newgen Imaging Systems (P) Ltd., Chennai, India
Printed in Great Britain
on acid-free paper by
Biddles Ltd., King's Lynn, Norfolk

ISBN 0–19–928708–2 978–0–19–928708–6

1 3 5 7 9 10 8 6 4 2

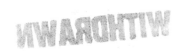

To Donald Davidson
In memory

Acknowledgments

Furthering a conversation between philosophy and psychoanalysis is a project that has engaged me for over thirty years. So many people have helped me with it in so many different ways—as teachers, analysts, friends, supervisors, philosophers, engaged interlocutors—that in expressing my gratitude both the starting and the stopping points are arbitrary.

I begin with psychoanalysis and the San Francisco Psychoanalytic Institute, a community that from the beginning of my work there was as eager to open its doors to the outside as I was to learn what I knew I could find only inside it. In particular I thank Drs Suzanne Gassner, Adrienne Applegarth, Maurice Marcus, Robert Wallerstein, and Joe Weiss. I should add that the patients I saw during my period of training, some of whom make an entrance here, of course much disguised, were an invaluable source of insight, not only into other minds but also into my own.

In philosophy I am grateful above all to Donald Davidson.

Sadly, Donald, Adrienne, and Joe are all now gone. But they live on in this book, and I hope would not be unhappy with the forms their presence takes.

Charles Altieri, Philip Edberg, Charles Fisher, Jeff Malpas, Richard Moran, Georges Rey, Barry Smith, and Barry Stroud all generously took time to read various parts of the manuscript. I have profited greatly from their comments, which is not to say that they ever did or will now agree with what I say.

In more daily ways, there are many others who have inspired and sustained me, in particular my daughter, Rachel Cavell.

Several of the chapters in this volume were originally published in some form elsewhere. I thank the various journals for permission to use them.

'Keeping Time: Remembering, Repeating, and Working Through' was first published as 'Keeping Time: Freud on the Temporality of Mind', in M. Levine (ed.), *The Analytic Mind* (London: Routledge, 1999).

'Triangulation: The Social Character of Thinking' is a revision of 'Triangulation: One's Own Mind and Objectivity', *International Journal of Psychoanalysis*, 79/3 (1998).

'On Judgment' is a revision of 'The Social Character of Thinking', *Journal of the American Psychoanalytic Association*, 51/3 (2003).

'Irrationality and Self-Transcendence' first appeared as 'Reason and the Gardener' in L. E. Hahn (ed.), *Philosophy of Donald Davidson* (The Library of Living Philosophers 27; Chicago: Open Court, 1999).

'Freedom and Understanding' is a revision of 'Freedom and Forgiveness', *International Journal of Psychoanalysis*, 84/3 (2003).

Contents

Introduction

Freud may not have discovered the unconscious, but he was the first to map psychological space. As such is he honored in the now old-fashioned phrase 'depth psychology'. But the space Freud explored is not only vertical; in it there are large, fairly stable structures of memory, habit, ideas, and structures that erode, shift, and are more or less responsive to ongoing experience; bewilderingly many paths along which thoughts and feelings are linked; and vistas just glimpsed at the edge of the frame.

This space has turned out to be so rich, so important in explaining behavior and in determining what it is like to be a particular person— her 'subjectivity'—that there has been a tendency in psychoanalysis to lose sight of the fact that we are animals in a real, physical world, equipped to deal with and to register what endangers us there and what helps us thrive. Through this book runs the theme that psychological space demands physical space; that the inner world is embedded in, and fabricated from, interactions between world and mind.

In an earlier book, *The Psychoanalytic Mind: From Freud to Philosophy*, (Cavell 1993), I was concerned with the implications for psychoanalysis of a particular contemporary theory of meaning that takes off from Wittgenstein and Davidson. I there distinguished two conflicting strains in psychoanalytic thought: one sees the mind as self-contained; the other claims that mind arises only within an interpersonal field, in a real material world that the subjects share, and come to know they share. This second position frames my reflections in this book as well. After setting it up, I turn my attention to themes in moral philosophy: the nature of the 'subject', agency, free will, and self-knowledge.

By 'subject' I mean someone who recognizes herself as an 'I', as having her own peculiar perspective; a subject is an agent who is able to be self-reflective, and to assume responsibility for herself and for some of her actions. The phrase 'becoming a subject' might suggest an exercise in developmental psychology. That is not my project, though I do make an argument that appeals to development in the chapter on triangulation.

I am inquiring, more generally, into the conditions, both developmental and conceptual, on which we can think in the first-person, and attribute a first person, subjective, view to others. I maintain that any discussion of what it is to be a human 'self' or 'subject' must acknowledge four ideas that are central to psychoanalysis: first, much mental functioning is unconscious, not necessarily through repression; second, memory takes different forms, which carry with them different degrees of conscious awareness; third, the degree of consciousness is often dictated by unconscious, defensive processes, summoned into play against pain and anxiety; and, finally, the past informs the present, often in ways of which we are unaware and over which we lack direct control.

Since I will be calling on these ideas throughout the book, I introduce them in 'Neuroscience, Psychoanalysis, and Memory', showing the ample support they receive from contemporary neuroscience. Together, the first three chapters are about memory, anxiety, and time. The second chapter is devoted to anxiety because of the role it plays in defensive behavior, and because it particularly manifests the complex relation between psychological space and the external world that I spoke of earlier. Freud's last revisionary paper, 'Inhibitions, Symptoms, and Anxiety' (Freud 1926), returned to the external world the importance in psychological life that he had given it in his earliest works. 'Keeping Time' reviews Freud's changing thoughts about memory, and the trio of inter-related concepts that he calls remembering, repeating (a certain failure of remembering), and working through (working a memory or a bit of learning through the fabric of one's mind and character as a whole). I discuss several ways in which psychoanalysts now attempt to explain neurotic repetition without hypothesizing, as Freud did, a basic instinct that is opposed to life.

The next three chapters are explicitly about the subject, and about first-person, propositional thought. 'Triangulation: The Social Character of Thinking' argues the interpersonal view of the mind alluded to above. 'On Judgment' elaborates Freud's idea of 'the reality principle' as in effect containing an analysis of the necessary conditions for propositional thought. I criticize attempts by psychoanalysts, notably Melanie Klein and Wilfred Bion, to derive such thought from fantasies. In 'Self-Reflections' I claim that investigations into the nature of the self that, like Descartes's, do not consider the background conditions for being able to think thoughts such as 'I am thinking' or 'I believe that *p*' are bound to give us a peculiar idea of selfhood. One can take neither the capacity for self-reference, nor the unity of the self, as given; such unity as there is comes about through processes of integration. In this context I consider Harry Frankfurt's idea of integrity as whole-hearted caring, which I argue is unsatisfactory, and that because it neglects the roles of other people and an openness to reality in the integrating process.

'Self-Reflections' is a hinge essay that also begins to address the issues of freedom and self-knowledge. 'Irrationality and Self-Transcendence' takes up a certain model of irrationality, exploring its implications for wilfully changing the person one is. 'Freedom and Understanding' argues that there are no conditions of a metaphysical nature that can rule out freedom, though various conditions of the sort with which psychoanalysts are familiar may partially erode the capacity for choice. In 'Valuing Emotions' I claim that emotions are quintessentially sub-jective states that are also intersubjective in important respects. As this chapter begins to discuss the many ways in which, with regard to the emotions in particular, one can fail to know one's own mind, it serves as a prelude to the final chapter, 'Self-Knowledge and Self-Discovery'. There I discuss the phenomenon of first-person authority, the Cartesian ocular model of introspection, and the relations between attitudes one can take toward oneself from a third-person perspective, and from a first-person perspective. These final chapters explicitly articulate the idea that one cannot hive off the subjective aspects of a person from those that are objective. A subject is a creature who can be seen both from a third-person and from a first-person point of view, and who can take both perspectives on herself. In turn, a view of another person that is objective about her must acknowledge that she has a first-person point of view.

Each of these topics deserves a book to itself. I hope that I never-theless say enough about them to show some of their interrelations, and their connections with psychoanalysis.

The Appendix is addressed primarily to psychoanalysts. It makes observations of a general sort about the concepts of knowledge, truth, and certainty, turning then to epistemological worries that psycho-analysts have raised in connection particularly with the clinical situation.

The direction of influence between philosophy and psychoanalysis goes both ways. As a theory concerned with what it is to be a person, with (as a matter of practice) enlarging the scope in which we act in some sense freely, and with self-knowledge, psychoanalysis can learn from philosophy, since that is where these themes are most thoughtfully engaged. In return, philosophical treatments of them demand, I believe, acknowledgment of some of the basic claims of psychoanalysis.

Between the two disciplines there is a large area of overlap, and obviously many differences, one of which is that in philosophy and the hard sciences the particular enters chiefly by way of instance and example, whereas in both its theory and its practice psychoanalysis must honor the fact that no two human beings are more than roughly alike. Freud has sometimes been criticized for assuming that there is such a thing as human nature, or a set of generalizations that can be made about all people at all times. I am not sure he does assume that. He certainly believes that major upheavals in culture can change what we have taken to be the natural and universal. (Think of *Totem and Taboo* and *Civilization and its Discontents*.) But, in any case, though psychoanalysis does often make sweeping generalizations about development, it does not generalize about 'the subject'; it takes each of us to be unique in ways that must shape whatever sort of 'science' about us there can be. Should psychoanalysis abandon that perspective, as it would be doing if, for instance, it decided that mind-talk could be thoroughly replaced with talk about neural circuitry, psycho-analysis would be dead. But, far from moving in that direction, analysts are increasingly aware just how complex the variables are that affect what each of us feels, thinks, or says to her analyst, and the particular analytic relationship itself.

Psychoanalysis is then, and must be, a peculiar 'science', as is reflected in the fact that 'psychoanalysis' refers at once to a theory of the mind, a mode of clinical practice, and a theory about that practice. Perhaps this peculiarity is one of the sources of the dismay it so often arouses. Though I believe there are also others.

For a long time a number of philosophers, interestingly more in Great Britain than in America, have known that their philosophical interests tied into psychoanalysis. From Great Britain one thinks of Stuart Hampshire, Ludwig Wittgenstein, John Wisdom, Richard Wollheim, Alasdair MacIntyre, David Pears, James Hopkins, Sebastian Gardner, David Snelling; from the United States and Canada: Herbert Fingarette (whose work has in my opinion been insufficiently appreciated), Richard Kuhns, Stanley Cavell, Jonathan Lear, Jerome Neu, Donald Davidson, Ronald de Sousa, Adolph Grunbaum (in scorn).

In person, a great many other philosophers have told me of their own experience as analysands, or have expressed interest in the subject. Often a philosopher will make a promising but undeveloped allusion to psychoanalysis. For example, Bernard Williams (1995: 202) writes:

A non-moralized, or less moralized, psychology uses the categories of meaning, reasons and value, but leaves it open, or even problematical, in what way moral reasons and ethical values fit with other motives and desires.... Thucydides and (I believe) the tragedians, among the ancient writers, had such a psychology; and so, in the modern world, did Freud.

Williams does not elaborate.

But all these philosophers are exceptions: neither in Great Britain nor in the United States has philosophy been much affected by psychoanalysis. One reason may be that Freud burdened his central theme, the unconscious workings of the mind, with a complex and unwieldy theory, many parts of which no longer bear up. Another may have to do with the fact that Freud was a strange mixture of clinician, scientist, philosopher, and brilliant writer. If, like the philosopher Colin McGinn (1999), one reads Freud primarily as an intellectual figure, ignoring the extent to which he was continually amending his own observations and theories, and not investigating the contemporary evidence for those of Freud's claims that are empirical, one will indeed find much to complain about.

Further, though his daily work consisted in listening to and making sense of stories, Freud could not help making far-reaching pronouncements (about the fundamental principles at work not only in the mind but in the universe, for example), some of which were at best purely speculative, at worst, absurd.

Many years after completing graduate work in philosophy I decided that to make my forays into psychoanalysis honest I needed some formal education in the matter. Full training at an institute accredited by the American Psychoanalytic Association, which perhaps for not very good reasons was what I wanted, involved taking on and completing several analytic cases, in addition to having one's own psychoanalysis. (There were and are a number of fine institutes that are not under the umbrella of the APA, often because they do not wish to be. Their requirements for graduation are different.) And in those days one could not treat patients unless one was a medical doctor, in particular a psychiatrist. So I became a Research Candidate at the Columbia Psychoanalytic Institute for Training and Research, meaning that I took courses, but not patients.

Some twenty years later I had moved to Berkeley; the rules of the APA had changed; and I decided I wanted clinical experience. I enrolled as a candidate at the San Francisco Psychoanalytic Institute and graduated from their Committee on Research and Special Training (CORST) program.

I should say that, though I sometimes draw on clinical experience to illustrate a point, I make no case for psychoanalysis as a valuable therapy. It will perhaps become clear, however, why I think it is.

PART I
Preliminary Remarks on Memory and Mind

I

Neuroscience, Psychoanalysis, and Memory

And so we ought not to fear in love, as in everyday life, the future alone, but even the past, which often comes to life for us only when the future has come and gone—and not only the past which we discover after the event but the past which we have long kept stored within ourselves and suddenly learn how to interpret.

(Marcel Proust, *The Rembrance of Things Past*)

Not long ago many of America's best artists, writers, and intellectuals were on the couch. Sought after by the most prestigious medical schools for the most prestigious positions, psychoanalysts could charge virtually what they wanted to patients who would sometimes wait months or years for the privilege of tying up an indefinite amount of money, time, and energy. Freud was not merely an important figure but, as W. H. Auden said, a whole climate of opinion, riding high on a wave of honor that carried him well into the 1980s.

For many reasons the crest has broken. Psychoanalysis has been attacked on every conceivable ground. It has been argued that its theory of the mind is baseless, or riddled with contradictions; that the changes Freud made over time in his own theories, often trumpeted by his fans as testimony to his openness of mind, served rather to get him out of some intellectual muddle into which his penchant for grandiose system building had sunk him in the first place; that psycho-analytic therapy does not work, or at least no better than many other much less costly and time-consuming forms of 'treatment', including religion and hand holding; that many of the events Freud reported in his case histories were fabrications; that Freud the man lacked integrity. In a scathing assault on Freud published in 1993 in the *New York Review of Books*, Frederick Crews, a professor of English, wrote that psychoanalysis has 'proved to be an indifferently successful method and vastly inefficient method of removing neurotic symptoms', and that 'Freud's doctrine has been faring no better, in scientifically respectable quarters, as a cluster of propositions about the Mind' (Crews 1993: 55).

About the second, at least, Crews is simply mistaken. Take Freud's most important thesis, that much mental functioning is unconscious, and kept out of consciousness by anxiety and defense against anxiety. Contemporary research amply supports it, along with such other important Freudian propositions as that childhood catastrophes reverberate in the adult mind, causing pathological ways of thinking and behaving; that memory has different ways of working, many of which are unconscious; and that anxiety misunderstood fixes us neurotically to the past. With Freud the Wordsworthian child, trailing clouds of glory, is gone. In her place is a child who, in D.W.Winnicott's memorable words, is falling forever, fragmenting into bits and pieces, a child who repeatedly plays abandonment and return. Even in the best of cases, defenses are brought into play that over time block perception, inhibit desire, and confound self-knowledge; at worst, they threaten life itself. It is a love story Freud tells, but one filled with catastrophe. If the human creature is peculiarly gifted with imagination and fantasy, we are also peculiarly susceptible to variations on the themes of love and loss; to self-deception, fantastic fears, false memories, and grand illusions, which color the present and hold us captive to the past.

I begin with the unconscious, which will quickly lead to memory, not surprisingly since without memory there could be no mind at all. We would not be able to perceive this object *as* a tree, this event *as* a storm; there could be no such thing as re-cognition; no awareness of something as threatening pain, or promising pleasure; no learning from experience. Adam Zeman (2002: 181) writes: 'Our knowledge of the world pervades perception. We are always seeking after meaning. Try *not* deciphering a road sign, or erasing the face of the man in the moon. What we see resonates in the memory of what we have seen; new experience always percolates through the old, leaving a hint of its flavor as it passes. We live, in this sense, in a "remembered present".' The vicissitudes of memory are then the vicissitudes of experience, and mind. 'The' unconscious is not an absence of mind, but, in the case of repression, a particular way of holding something in, or out of, mind.

We will turn, then, to the emotions, which psychoanalysis has always known are the heart of mind, and the matter of every psychoanalysis.

The Unconscious, Memory, and Neuroscience

Gerald Edelman (1992: 145) writes: 'The postulation of an unconscious is a central binding principle of Freud's psychological theories. Since his time, ample evidence has accumulated from the study of neurosis, hypnotism, and parapraxes to show that his basic theses about the action of the unconscious were essentially correct.'

If this is so, why is the idea of the unconscious still resisted? One answer is that we still don't like it. As Freud himself said, the idea that we are much less in our own control than we think we are is frightening. Another is that the 'Freudian' unconscious carries with it the greatest burden of now outdated psychoanalytic theory. For example: Freud thought 'the unconscious' was a single system, possessing its own mental laws. Sometimes he equated the unconscious with the 'id', sometimes with instinct, or drive. He even suggested that 'mental processes are in themselves unconscious'. While contemporary studies vindicate the ideas of both unconscious mental processes and repression, they suggest that Freud's idea of a single unconscious system should be revised, that instead there are many kinds of unconscious processes that serve different functions (Westen 1999: 1062). And similarly with memory. Only twenty years or so ago, cognitive psychologists assumed, contra Freud, that most cognitive processes are conscious. Memory was believed to consist in bringing thoughts into short-term memory, a term that is now replaced by the more comprehensive 'working memory'. The distinction between short-term and long-term memory implied that at least some memories in the second system must be unconscious; but the distinction was not explored. Instead, researchers assumed 'that thoughts (and presumably motives and emotions . . .) could only influence action to the extent that they were perceived, registered, consciously processed, and then retrieved into short-term memory (*alias* consciousness)' (Westen 1999: 1065).

The current consensus is that, as there are many kinds of unconscious mental processes, so also are there multiple memory systems, each obeying different rules of operation, which interact to produce our subjective experience of remembering. Schacter (1999: 148–59) writes:

Our normally seamless awareness of episodes from our personal pasts and knowledge of the world masks a great deal of underlying complexity. Remembering one's wedding depends on a different brain network than knowing where a bar of soap can be found. Recognizing a submarine requires different neural machinery than recognizing a spider. Each of these types of knowledge depends on the integrity of specific constellations of underlying brain structures and processes.

The old distinction between short-term and long-term memory barely scratches the surface. Taxonomies of memory abound, some of which cut across each other. Since they will undoubtedly change over the coming decades, it is not important to get all the distinctions straight, but to notice how many kinds of memory there are.

Most neuroscientists agree in distinguishing two broad systems. First, there are memories of the events in our lives, and the knowledge of the world we have gained through them. Typically these memories can be retrieved when the situation calls for it, which is why they are called explicit, also sometimes declarative, meaning that you can say what it is you are remembering. ('Explicit' and 'declarative' are often used as synonyms in this context, but I will shortly draw a distinction between them.) Explicit memory includes things like remembering the day your grandmother became ill, and what you did then; or remembering *that* Thomas Jefferson was the third president of the United States; or *that* the Galapagos islands were important in Darwin's developing evolutionary theory. Explicit memory is essentially subject-ive, available to your awareness, and only to yours. It is, we might say, first person and narrative in character. Implicit memory, on the other hand, is often not conscious, verbal, nor first person. If the memory is explicit and declarative, you are reminded of the trip, where you were going, whom you were with. You also remember *that* you were frightened, but you are not necessarily frightened now. With implicit memory, present emotion kicks in. The taste of the madeleine does not merely recall the past to Marcel, it evokes it emotionally now; bending down to tie his shoe suddenly reminds him of an incident with his grandmother some time before she died, and he weeps for her for the first time.

The 'explicit self' refers to things we consciously know about ourselves, the 'implicit self' to all the aspects of ourselves that are not immediately available to consciousness. Both may be influenced similarly or differently at any one point. For example, a mild put-down may only be registered and stored in explicit memory. But a flagrant insult, registered explicitly, 'might lead to the arousal of emotion systems that then also store aspects of the experience implicitly' (LeDoux 2002: 29).

Implicit memory includes memories for various skills, habits, and procedures that we have acquired through experience. This particular type of memory is therefore called *procedural*. (The hippocampus is essential to explicit memory, but not to implicit memory.) Watching the child take up the cup in both hands so that he will not spill it, I infer that he remembers learning how to do that; but this is a memory he need not consciously have. Knowing how to pick up the cup, or ride a bike, is an instance of *procedural* memory; it is a *knowing how* rather than a *knowing that*. (Familiarity with human practices, like using particular tools in particular, culturally determined ways, which Heidegger thought precedes and sets the stage for language learning, might be considered procedural knowledge.)

Not only is conscious reflection unnecessary to procedural know-ledge, it may even get in the way: if you think about your backhand in the middle of a tennis game, or of what your fingers are doing while you play the Chopin F minor Étude, you may skid to a halt altogether. Sometimes people can say how they carry out such procedures, but often, even as adults, we cannot. I could show, but not tell, a child how to tie his shoe.

Another kind of implicit memory of special importance to psy-choanalysis is called *associative*. As its name indicates, it involves the ways in which memories are organized, namely, along pathways that are associative and idiosyncratic: 'tea' calls to my mind not 'coffee', nor 'beverage', but a visit to my grandmother's country house. Implicit, associative memories connect to other unconscious memories by links that would not be obviously relevant to a 'rational' eye. (We recall Freud's early hypothesis (1896: 1) that hysterical symp-toms do not arise from real experiences alone, but from memories of earlier experiences that are awakened in association to it. It is their specificity and their enmeshment in a particular narrative that help account, I suggest, for the 'subjectivity', the uniqueness, 'the feel' of one's experience.[1]

The psychoanalytic principle of free association obviously rests on the idea of associative networks. Let your mind go, in a relaxed and safe environment, and it will travel along paths different from those you take when your thinking is problem-solving and purposive, as when you ask yourself, 'What would be the kindest way to tell Mary she has failed her audition?' or 'Do I really want to go to Paris in June, since that means that I couldn't go to Mary's wedding?' Freud believed that associative thinking is distinctive of what he called primary process thought, thought that is guided by wish and developmentally more primitive than reality-oriented, 'secondary process' thought; but it now seems rather that all thought, memory, and perception may move along associative networks (Westen 1999: 1071; Brakel et al. 2000).

The explicit/implicit distinction cuts through that between short-term and long-term memory, as well as through a distinction between *episodic* and *semantic* memory. Episodic memory concerns the specific context of an experienced event, including the time and place of its occurrence. Semantic memories, on the other hand, are acquired during an event but are stored separately from the memory of the event itself. Semantic memory is 'a network of associations and concepts that underlies our basic knowledge of the world—word meanings, categories, facts and propositions, and the like'. Studies of amnesiac patients show that semantic memory can remain partially intact even when episodic memory is entirely dysfunctional. For example: Gene, who suffered a severe head injury during a motor-cycle accident, cannot recall either the accident, or any other specific episode from any time in his life. So far as he knows he has no past, nor does he think about the future. But though he does not remember going to school, he knows where he went to school, that he worked at a certain plant before his accident, that he owned two motorcycles and a car, and so on. He can also describe in detail

---

[1] Implicit memory may account for the uncanny experience of *déja vu*, the feeling of having already lived through an event that is presumably occurring for the first time. According to one theory, *déja vu* occurs when a fragment of a memory is activated by a present situation but cannot be remembered explicitly; so what is happening for the first time seems to be happening 'again' (Schacter 1996).

what is involved in changing the tire, even though he cannot recall changing one himself (Schacter 1996: 150–1).

The sensory aspects of things we experience, their value to us as 'good' or 'bad', the associations we have made between them and other things and events in the world, are all a part of semantic memory. Just what the relations are between semantic and episodic memory is not clear, though it is agreed that they are different systems, separated in the brain, and that semantic memory predates the development of episodic memory (Payne et al. 2002).

The distinctions above refer to different properties of mental events, and so to some extent, as I said earlier, they cut across each other. The declarative/procedural distinction refers to the type of knowledge (facts versus skills), whereas the explicit/implicit distinction refers to the way this knowledge is expressed and stored (with or without conscious awareness). Both declarative and procedural knowledge can be either explicit and conscious, or implicit and unconscious. Declarative knowledge is explicit, as when you consciously recall an event from childhood, say, or implicit and unconscious, as when you fail to remember a painful event, or distort it as a way of warding off feelings of anxiety. Procedural knowledge is explicit when you are aware of using a particular skill, implicit when it is caught up in the unconscious use of a mechanism that wards off a painful feeling.

What psychoanalysts call defenses to regulate painful affect presumably involve implicit, unconscious procedures (Westen 2002: 79). They are remnants of the ways in which, without thinking, one initially dealt with the painful situation. (You blamed someone else when you were feeling accused; you turned to stone when your feelings were hurt; you responded with contempt when you were feeling belittled or left out.) Thereafter they are unconsciously summoned into play in situations that seem to threaten a similar wound. Now they are automatic and not under voluntary control, hence not permitting much flexibility in deciding what action will be most appropriate for solving a problem.[2]

[2] Controlled procedures, on the other hand, call for declarative knowledge, which must be conscious while one is performing the procedure. The capacity for declarative knowledge matures approximately in the fifth year, which means that before then the child has little control over how what he has learned will affect his behavior.

Emotional Memory

Some researchers think we may need to posit emotional memory as a distinctive system to which some of the earlier distinctions are applicable. Joseph LeDoux concentrates on fear, which he suggests we consider as a system not for experiencing fear but for detecting danger and responding to it with defensive behavior. Much of what he says about fear may generalize, he believes, to other emotions.

Why the emphasis on fear? For one thing, it is necessary to survival. For another, it pervades human experience in the forms of apprehension, anxiety, shyness, dread, shame, and guilt. Philosophers like Kierkegaard, Heidegger, Sartre, and Binswanger place *angst* or anxiety at the center of human experience; in their view our integrity as persons is a function of how we handle anxiety. Child psychologists agree that fear of abandonment is fundamental to childhood and pervasively influential in human behavior long afterwards.

With a few other writers, LeDoux distinguishes emotional processes from feeling. His view is that 'a subjective emotional experience, like the feeling of being afraid, results when we become consciously aware that an emotion system of the brain, like the defense system, is active' (LeDoux 1998: 268). The emotional meaning of a stimulus can begin to be appraised by the brain before it has made its way into conscious perception; that is, the brain may evaluate something as threatening— 'bad'—before the person herself knows exactly what the stimulus is and what is threatening about it.

LeDoux also distinguishes between emotional responses that are direct, not mediated by cognition, and those that are. From stimulus, say a large spider, to fear, there are two neural pathways, both converging in the amygdala, the part of the brain that causes visceral and behavioral responses. One path takes 'the low road', bypassing cognition and thought entirely; the other goes through the thalamus and then to the neocortex, the thinking part of the brain, whose job is to prevent an inappropriate response.

An animal that fears fire because it has been burned by fire is responding appropriately to a real danger. But stimuli occur in contexts. It is the hippocampus that provides the amygdala with information about the context of the emotional experience, allowing data from multiple memory systems to be unified into what may become, for a creature who can tell one, a coherent story. It is the context, provided by episodic memory, that makes human memory autobiographical, locating memories in space and time: 'This happened then, after I'd done that, when you and I were on our way to there.' 'The context is, in other words, a psychological construction, a kind of memory created on the spot, about the various factors that constitute an emotional situation' (LeDoux 2002: 216).

We recall that Freud quickly abandoned his assumption that memory is a veracious record of the past, for a view of memory as a construction. A plea, however, for the truth of memory. Though I may have edited and embroidered them, my memories of the train wreck we were in, your birthday party last year, dancing at my wedding, may record events that truly happened, and that you and others who were there may remember in much the way I do. The details of our stories will differ. I remember them in ways peculiar to me, and, were I to tell them in a story, the story would be different from yours of the same events. There would be different details, different emphases, but of the same events.

Implicit emotional memories and explicit memories of emotional experiences meet in working memory, where potentially they can be modified into a new explicit long-term memory that is not emotion-ally disturbing; for, once in working memory, thoughts can modify activity back down the hierarchy. But, because of the gap between our advanced cognitive capacities and the older emotional and motivational systems, 'downward causation' is difficult, as anyone who has survived a successful psychoanalysis knows. Furthermore, working memory can itself be disturbed by chronic or extreme stress. And, finally, the conditions that lead to a weakened ability to form explicit memories and to regulate fear by reflection and reasoning can also magnify fear reactions and enhance the ability to store implicitly information about traumatic or stressful situations (LeDoux 2002). Thus stress impairs explicit memory while it enhances implicit emotional memories (Payne et al. 2002).

How far back do emotional memories go? Apparently, very far. Researchers have concluded that the infant mind registers affective experiences before it can use symbols, and that the child's pre-verbal, affectively colored experiences continue to exert an influence through-out life, particularly on his or her interpersonal relations (Stern 1983).

One of the major differences between rats and human beings is that we use symbols, tell stories, see the same thing under different descriptions—the man you just met *as* a writer, a spendthrift, the former lover of your friend Mary, and so on. The number of ways in which any of us can see a particular thing or event is potentially infinite, and so, therefore, are the changes that can be rung on our perceptions, beliefs, and emotions. Language is not necessary for all emotional states, but for a great many it is, since it is language that allows us to articulate the world more finely, and hence to have a wider, more finely articulated array of emotional responses. It is language, and the concepts that come with it, that make possible sophisticated emotions like shame and guilt. For us the world holds both more joys and more terrors than it can for other creatures: Bach; the fear of dying; Balanchine; the emotionally difficult task of taking in that you were an unwanted and hated child.

Put our gifts for language and for aspect-seeing together with the fact that the mind moves along associative as well as logical pathways, and we understand how free association may lead from a seemingly unimportant thought into a warren of deep-seated, emotionally charged memories.

Repression, Recall, and Reconstruction

Freud called those thoughts and memories that are out of conscious awareness for a reason, namely, to avoid unpleasure, 'repressed'. His earliest theories pictured the mind in terms of conscious and unconscious functioning; but this did not make room for what he found to be the clinical fact that the act of censorship is itself unconscious. This was one reason why he introduced the 'structural view' of the mind in terms of ego, id, and super-ego, where 'ego' names a set of conscious and unconscious functions, one of which is to censor, in the absence of conscious awareness, potentially dangerous perceptions and emotions.

On the face of it the idea of unconscious censorship is self-contradictory; for in order to hide a painful feeling or perception from itself, the mind must know what it wants to hide. Thus we would seem to be led to an infinite series of censors, each monitoring the one before. For this reason Sartre argued, like many philosophers after him, that the idea of repression is incoherent: however many layers of consciousness we add, censor and censored must end up on the same side of the divide; it is the same 'self', the same 'I', that both knows and does not know.

But these arguments assume that consciousness has always the same— what shall I say?—degree; and assume as well a unitary; motivational system rather than a multiplicity of systems connected to each other in a variety of ways (Tyson 2000). Where Freud thought of repression as an absolute barrier, current evidence suggests we might better think of it is as an inhibitory process that has varying degrees (Westen 2002: 89). Here is another way of putting it that will make more sense once I have talked about 'the self' (Chapter 6): not all the activities of the mind are ones for which 'I' can speak.

Neisser was the first cognitive psychologist to use the information-processing model of the mind as a way of conceptualizing defenses against painful experiences. Perception and memory, are processes that take place in time, traveling a route of which explicit consciousness is a relatively late stage. In the earliest, incoming stimuli are broken up into the sorts of chunks that 'episodic memory' refers to, and stored under categories like 'spider', 'thing that bites', 'comforting figure', 'mother', 'blue'. Neisser calls the primitive stage of processing pre-attentive. How the information is sorted is open to emotional influence, such that we may avoid construction in certain areas (Neisser 1967).

This 'information' model fits with the work on the emotions described above according to which affective evaluation does not require consciousness or cognitive awareness. Without knowing it, we learn unconsciously to associate aspects of situations or other people with pleasant or unpleasant feelings. As a result, we can respond, also unconsciously, to cues that lead us to avoid situations or people who match the prototype of the earlier experiences (Westen 1999: 1074–5). Well-known studies with a tachistoscope—an instrument that flashes subliminal messages on a screen as it tests visceral and behavioral responses—are best explained by positing a motivated failure to register consciously a perception that has been registered unconsciously. For example: the subject is shown pictures designed to arouse disgust or conflicted feelings. He denies having seen the pictures, though his body indicates that he has (Shevrin et al. 1996).

Other studies show that we can willfully suppress the memory of an unwanted past experience, and that the suppression becomes more thorough the longer it is maintained (Anderson et al. 2004). Yet others support the idea of perceptual defense, a screening of sensory input that selects which percepts will be further processed into consciousness (Erdelyi 1974). Solms and Solms have shown that patients who have suffered massive injuries of some sort can consciously deny or 'neglect' their injuries while knowing of them unconsciously, and that this neglect is evidently motivated (Kaplan-Solms and Solms 2000: 157–67).

The idea of repressed memories of childhood sexual abuse, which some analysts prefer to describe as dissociated rather than repressed, has elicited the harshest response from Freud's critics. Undoubtedly some such 'memories' are fabricated; but here too there is a convincing body of evidence, the strongest of which comes from a study of women who had been treated in hospital for genital injury resulting from sexual molestation when they were children. Seventeen years after their documented abuse, 38 percent of them could not remember the event, even though many of these women reported later incidents of sexual abuse. The suggestion that they might have merely forgotten is implausible: having one's genitals sufficiently damaged to require hospitalization is not the sort of memory that simply erodes with time (Westen 1999: 1077–80).

Does trauma lead to a heightened memory of the traumatic event, or to 'forgetting'? Both. Nietzsche speaks of what he calls 'active oblivion' as a 'concierge', whose role is to 'shut temporarily the doors and windows of consciousness' in order to make room for peace and order. But punishment, trauma, the inducement of guilt, do not allow the concierge to work. 'There is perhaps nothing more terrible in man's earliest history than his mnemotechnics. A thing is branded on the memory to make it stay there; only what goes on hurting will stick' (Nietzsche 1956: 192). As if in a nod to Nietzsche, LeDoux (1996: 265) tells us that emotional memories are 'burned' into the amygdala's circuits, and cannot be erased. Yet at the same time, as I noted earlier, above, trauma can damage or shut down the part of the brain (the hippocampus) that is responsible for explicit, episodic, memory.

Freud seems to have been right, then, in claiming that trauma affects unconscious memory; that memories can date to early childhood; that childhood experiences reverberate through one's life, affecting how we perceive the world and what we do; that we may have little or no conscious recollection of an experience that has nevertheless left powerful, implicit, emotional memories; that we may unconsciously 'know' something without knowing that we do; that there is a motivated unknowing; and that present behavior can be out of touch with present reality through the work of what we might now call unconscious, procedural, memories that serve a defensive purpose.

Freud also claimed that unconscious memories can sometimes be recovered, and that recovering them can lead to the relief of symptoms. Do we have reason to think that either is true? Psychoanalysts answer, Yes. So does LeDoux (1996: 244):

Let's assume that it is indeed possible for a temporary period of trauma to lead to an amnesia for the experience. Can one later recover a memory of these events? ... if the hippocampus was completely shut down by the stress to the point where it had no capacity to form a memory during the event, then it will be impossible by any means to dredge up a conscious memory ... On the other hand, if the hippocampus was only partially affected, it may have participated in the formation of a weak and fragmented memory. Such memories will of necessity involve 'filling in the blanks'. . .

And again (1966: 263)

Freud's psychoanalytic theory and the various conditioning theories all assume that anxiety is the result of traumatic learning experiences that foster the establishment of anxiety-producing long-term memories. In this sense, psychoanalytic and conditioning theories have drawn similar conclusions about the origin of anxiety. However, the two kinds of theory lead to two different therapeutic approaches. Psychoanalysis seeks to make the patient conscious of the origins of inner conflict, whereas behavior therapy ... tries to rid the person of the symptoms ... through various forms of conditioning.

Though the amygdala's emotional memories may never be erased, their effects can be modified if a narrative context is recovered or created that gives the stimulus a new meaning. Therapy 'does not erase the memory that ties fear reactions to trigger stimuli ... [it] rather prevents the stimuli from unleashing the fear reaction' (LeDoux 1996: 146). In short, one can become aware that alarm signals have been set off, and appraise their appropriateness. Instead of the mind's being flooded with a feeling that 'this is happening now', one can recognize that the feeling belongs to something that happened in the past. Automaticity yields to control.

This is what psychoanalytic therapy has always been about: separating past from present; mending time; amplifying the degree of freedom with which one responds to difficult situations. In *Constructions in Analysis*, Freud (1937: 257) writes: 'It is familiar ground that the work of analysis aims at inducing the patient to give up the repressions (*using the word in the widest sense*) belonging to his early development and to replace them by reactions of a sort that would correspond to a psychically mature condition' (emphasis added).

Implicit emotional memories are 'recovered' when the affect is consciously felt. One of the goals of psychoanalytic therapy is to provide a situation of safety in which old emotions can be re-experienced, which is why psychoanalysts make such a fuss about transference—that is, the patient's casting the analyst in the role of a familiar figure in a traumatic, past relationship. To be modified the emotional memory has to be lived, which is why the transforming self-discovery in psychoanalysis is necessarily painful, not merely intellectually knowing *that* your mother repeatedly shamed you, or made you feel you were a burden, but feeling those feelings now. How do we know this is what the patient was feeling *then*? We don't. But it doesn't matter. What *does* matter is what she is feeling *now*. Articulating this may lead her to the past, then return her to an understanding of how she frames the world in the present. An example: Marian is feeling anxious, and irritated. She is not sure herself what she feels, or why. Indeed, if she knew the one, she would know the other. Let us assume the following: she realizes that she was thinking for herself, 'for a change', and was feeling proud. But then she became alarmed because she thought I was angry. Assume also that I was not angry, and that she comes to agree that she had no good reason for thinking I was. Her irritation fades. But now she wonders: was this a simple misunderstanding of me, or one guided, misguided, by the past? She remembers how angry her father used to become when she acted independently. She sees that her beliefs, perhaps correct about her childhood father, inform her relations in the present. Now she is in position to be more attentive to what is going on, both in herself and in others.

All of us perceive the present in terms of the past, bring to our relationships an affective repertoire we learned earlier. But the neurotic's responses are more stereotypical; the stories he tells about himself in relation to other people are more skewed by anxiety, and defenses against anxiety. And these defenses affect what others see and feel in return, whose behavior may inadvertently reinforce the neurotic perceptions.

Psychotherapy aims, then, to focus conscious attention on a procedure that was never registered in consciousness—a meaning of 'making conscious the unconscious' quite different from what Freud had in mind (Westen 2002: 70). The hope is that one learns to become aware of the emotion before it sets the defensive behavior in action, which then allows for that flexibility of response that comes with explicit awareness. Freedom of the will, to which I return in a later chapter, comes, in part, with this flexibility, and this flexibility with language. LeDoux (1996: 197) tells us what we already know, that 'language radically alters the brain's ability to compare, contrast, discriminate, associate on-line, in real time, and to use such information to guide thinking and problem-solving'.

Both behavioral therapy and psychoanalysis may lead to greater discrimination and flexibility, LeDoux remarks. However, the neural roads taken may be different.

Extinction [behavioral] therapy may take place through a form of implicit learning involving the prefrontal-amygdala circuit, whereas psychoanalysis, with emphasis on conscious insight and conscious appraisals, may involve the control of the amygdala by explicit knowledge through the temporal lobe memory systems and other cortical areas involving conscious awareness . . . it is well known that the connections from the cortical areas to the amygdala are far weaker than the connections from the amygdala to the cortex. This may explain why it is so easy for emotional information to invade our conscious thoughts, but so hard for us to gain conscious control over our emotions. Psychoanalysis may be such a prolonged process because of this asymmetry. (LeDoux 1996: 265)

Psychoanalysts themselves say that whether emotional remembering leads to change depends on a number of factors, such as the extent to which the person has control over the memory and the degree to which the original affect is re-experienced. Sometimes, Westen (2002: 70) remarks, treatment may depend less on emotional recall 'than on understanding and altering associations and procedures, activated by certain experiences, which may be the only mnemonic residues . . .'.

This account of emotional memory raises puzzles that go to the heart of 'the talking cure'. How can we diminish the impact of a memory by giving it a verbal form it never had? If the narrative context is constructed, rather than remembered or reconstructed, how can it gear into emotional memory? In what form, if any, can such a memory—implicit and unconscious—be retrieved? How can words be so important in the relief of symptoms, the change of character?

The questions are familiar in the history of psychoanalysis. Frank (1969) speaks of the 'unrememberable and unforgettable'; Bollas (1987) of the 'unthought known'; Stern (1985: 71–2) of 'unformulated experience':

When a patient is finally able to think about a previously unaccepted part of life, seldom are fully formulated thoughts simply waiting to be discovered, ready for exposition. Instead, what is usually experienced is a kind of confusion—a confusion with newly appreciable possibilities . . . Unconscious clarity rarely underlies defense . . . 'Unformulated experience' is the label I have chosen to refer to mentation characterized by a lack of clarity and differentiation. Cognitions do not necessarily exist in the unformulated state, though, since the unformulated is a conglomeration not yet knowable in the separate and definable terms of language . . .

Schafer (1980) and Spence (1982) describe the analytic task as the patient's construction of a new life story.

Freud raised these questions himself, though in general he was inclined to conceive of mental content as articulate and in principle articulable. He assumed that perception is a sensory given, and that, when language comes along, it attaches to contents and perceptions that are already replete. In *Constructions in Analysis* Freud likens the analyst to the archaeologist: both wish to dig up a past that is preserved now as it then was—though the analyst works under more favorable conditions, since

he has at his disposal material which can have no counterpart in excavations, such as the repetitions of reactions dating from infancy and all that is indicated by the transference in connection with these repetitions . . . the excavator is dealing with destroyed objects of which large and important portions have quite certainly been lost, by mechanical violence, by fire and by plundering . . . The one and only course open is that of reconstruction, which for this reason can reach only a certain degree of probability. But it is different with

the psychical object whose early history the analyst is seeking to recover...
All of the essential elements are preserved; even things that seem completely
forgotten are present somehow and somewhere, and have merely been buried
and made inaccessible to the subject. (Freud 1937: 259–60)

   Freud vacillates between 'construction' and 'reconstruction'. The
analyst's task is 'to make out what has been forgotten from the traces
which it has left behind or, more correctly, to *construct* it'. Yet a few lines
later he refers to 'the analyst's work of construction, or, *if it is preferred,
of reconstruction* (Freud 1937: 259; emphasis added). In construction we
build something new; in reconstruction we try to build anew something that has to some degree and in some way been destroyed. So just
under the surface of Freud's rhetoric lie the questions: What do we
mean by 'remembering' as it takes place in a psychoanalysis? Is the tale
that is told an old tale, or a new tale, or perhaps a mixture of both? What
do we mean by a psychoanalytic interpretation? Is self-discovery a
finding, or a making? I will be coming at this last question from several
different directions throughout this book.

   As for interpretation, Freud (1937: 261) says that 'the word applies to
something one does to some single element of the material, such as
an association or a parapraxis. It is a "construction" when one lays
before the subject of the analysis a piece of his early history that he has
forgotten'. Depending on the sort of memory in question, instead of
saying it was forgotten we might now say it was never known; or that it
was known implicitly and procedurally, not declaratively and explicitly.
What is constructed, or discerned, and then given words, is sometimes
a procedural rule, or an affective disposition that forms the background
against which one interprets the world. By dispositions I mean things
like the tendency to think one is being cheated, or that one has been
unfairly treated, or that one can do anything one wants with impunity;
or the tendency not to think before acting.

   I asked: How can we diminish the impact of a memory by giving it
a verbal form it never had? And how can words be so important in the
relief of symptoms, the change of character? One answer has to do with
the fact that, when the context of an image or a memory is changed, so
is its affective meaning. Here is a simple analogy. You show Marilyn
a close-up of a woman crying. Since the woman resembles Marilyn's
mother, the picture is affectively laden for her. She feels sad, perhaps
even guilty. Now you show her a larger picture in which the woman

is sitting in front of a birthday cake, at the center of a circle of people who are smiling and applauding. Marilyn's sadness disappears.

Since I wrote the words above I have learned of evidence from LeDoux's laboratory and elsewhere that supports a hypothesis about memory that has extremely interesting implications for psychoanalytic practice. According to the 'classical consolidation' theory of memory, articulated in Roman times in the work of Quintilian and taken up again in the beginning of the twentieth century, there is a period immediately following the reception of 'information' during which it is labile and can be perturbed, affecting the way it is stored and consolidated into an engram. Once consolidated, the information remains in the form in which it was stored, unless the memory is destroyed. It was believed that there is one consolidation process per engram.

Now there is evidence that the process of retrieval itself, or remembering, makes the memory labile. To be stored in memory it must now be consolidated again, that is, reconsolidated, in a new form. On the 'hard' version of this *reconsolidation* theory, there is a core memory that is not changed; on the 'soft' version, whatever you learn in the retrieval period goes back into long-term memory. The 'hard' version is contentious among neuroscientists, but the 'soft' version is accepted by all (Duvall 2005). The explicit clinical implication of this research is that the consolidation (or reconsolidation) of traumatic memories can be inhibited, say through the injection of certain chemicals. More broadly, the reconsolidation hypothesis gives us another way of understanding the therapeutic process Freud called *remembering* and *working through*, to which I turn in Chapter 3.

2
The Anxious Animal

The state of man: inconstancy, boredom, anxiety.

(Blaise Pascal, *Provincial Letters*)

Other animals experience fear. A particular form of anxious imagining may be unique to us. Perhaps it is this form of anxiety more than anything else that, to quote Philip Larkin in 'Days', 'Brings the priest and the doctor | In their long coats | Running over the fields.'

For continental philosophers like Kierkegaard, Heidegger, and Sartre, anxiety is the central problem of our lives. It is how we affectively register our acknowledgment of certain profoundly disturbing aspects of the human world, just those aspects that define our existence as specifically human beings, agents, subjects: that we act, and must, in the absence of signposts whose accuracy is guaranteed, on the basis of rules and principles whose interpretation is finally up to us; that our lives are contingent on things beyond our ken and control; that we are 'thrown' into a world to which our existence is irrelevant; that as subjects we have no choice but to make choice: we are inexorably free.

But we try to mask anxiety with 'idle talk' (Heidegger), or by treating ourselves as mere passive objects, moved by circumstance and the irresistible will of others (Sartre). In constructing an authentic human life—one in which one learns to become a responsible agent and to accept the conditions of human existence—anxiety is not to be eased or dispelled, but lived. (One reason self-knowledge is so hard to come by in such matters is that truth and error can look much alike. Behind the assumption that you and you alone are to blame for something may lie the fantasy that all the power is yours; yet denying all responsibility would be self-deception. The belief that if you think hard enough you can guarantee the success of your plan may hide the fantasy that you can or should be omniscient; yet acting without thought may be a strategy for avoiding a decision.)

Anxiety has come to be one of the central concepts also in psycho-analysis. While there is wide divergence in contemporary psychoanalytic techniques, analysts converge in treating the patient's affective experience, as contrasted with instinctual conflict, as an entry point for exploring unconscious meanings (Kernberg 1993). Anxiety has the importance it does because our attempts to get away from it are among the major sources of self-destructive behavior; we often respond to anxiety automatically rather than thoughtfully, and in ways that blunt perception. It is axiomatic among psychoanalysts that the patient will not unlearn these automatic responses until he can live with anxiety long enough to recognize and understand it. And we see many forms of pathology as rooted in anxieties that have to do with acknowledging the same existential facts about which continental philosophers speak.

One difference between the philosophical and the psychoanalytic accounts lies in the emphasis of the latter on development. While Heidegger writes eloquently about how we avoid acknowledging time and death, he does not set adult avoidances of anxiety in the context of childhood anxieties that leave their mark. All children experience anxiety around the possibilities of loss and abandonment; around conflicts between maintaining ties to the ones they love and exploring the world on their own. Particular traumatic situations involving these anxieties can inhibit the child from moving increasingly into a condition in which he can act as an agent, be more fully a subject, exercise choice, and accept responsibility.

Later, what can seem a perfectly normal, adult, 'existential' anxiety—say, the fear of death, or taking a new job—can be paralyzing because of its connections to unconscious or implicit memories of childhood traumas when one was truly too immature and vulnerable to master the anxiety on one's own. In these cases, therapy requires that the adult re-experience these earlier anxieties in a safe environment, learning as he does so that he is no longer so helpless as he was then; and also that, because of anxious imaginings, he has misapprehended what is going on in the present moment. He attributes meanings that are incorrect in relation to the present, and may miss others that are relevant. The task is to exchange not anxiety for idle talk, but paralyzing anxiety burdened with terrors that are no longer realistic for an anxiety one can tolerate, and understand, and manage.

In contemporary neurobiological theory, 'signal anxiety', to which I turn shortly, includes two important ideas. (1) An event that is in itself innocent can serve as a signal of danger, as in Pavlovian conditioning. We saw earlier how this might work in discussing implicit memory and procedural learning. (2) This signal can be set off in the absence of conscious awareness. We might think of signal anxiety as a subset of unconscious mental processes that function to warn the creature of an approaching danger (Wong 1999: 1817). This conception of signal anxiety is thoroughly congruent with Freud, for whom 'condensation', 'displacement', and the rewritings of memory specified the associative pathways of implicit processes.

Anxiety, then, has a temporal complexity that forms part of its very content. Some of this content is unconscious, not necessarily repressed, but implicit. When unconscious, it can motivate behaviors in relation to which the sufferer is not entirely an agent.

I want briefly to summarize the changes in Freud's thinking about anxiety, climaxing with his 1926 'Inhibitions, Symptoms, and Anxiety', and then go on to a fuller discussion of signal anxiety.

In his *Introductory Lectures on Psycho-Analysis*, Freud (1916: 404) had said that anxiety is at 'the very center of our interest in the problems of neurosis'. In such early writing 'anxiety' referred to a felt experience of dread or apprehension, accompanied by certain physiological reactions. Freud distinguished fear from anxiety in several ways, one of which, mentioned in the previous chapter, calls fear a response to a present and specific danger, anxiety a response to an imagined future.

Later Freud (1920: 12) linked anxiety to surprise: 'Anxiety describes a particular state of expecting the danger or preparing for it, even though it may be an unknown one. "Fear" requires a definite object of which to be afraid. "Fright", however, is the name we give to the state a person gets into when he has run into danger without being prepared for it; it emphasizes the factor of surprise.' Contemporary human and animal studies support Freud in showing that the sense of having some control, of being prepared for danger, can profoundly mitigate the amount of stress the creature experiences (Payne et al. 2002).

In this same passage Freud (1920: 12) suggests that anxiety defends against fright. 'There is something about anxiety that protects the subject against *actual* fright and so against fright neuroses.'

In his early work Freud understood anxiety in terms of his energic model of the mind: anxiety is what happens to libido when it is repressed: first repression, then anxiety as the transformation of libido under repression. Neurotics suffer from anxiety because they have repressed their sexual impulses. (Recall Peter Sellars's spoof of psychoanalysis in the 1962 version of Hollywood's *Lolita*, Quilty masquerading as the school psychiatrist who tells Humbert Humbert that Lolita's peculiar behavior is 'ze rrrezult of sexual rrrepression'.) Normal and neurotic anxiety were to be distinguished by the fact that the first corresponds to 'external' dangers, the second to ones that are 'internal'. In the second case the ego needs to defend itself against the id, which it does through primary repression, then with symptom formation. Phobic symptoms, for instance, replace an internal, instinctual danger with an external, perceptual one.

'Inhibitions, Symptoms, and Anxiety' (1926) announces a fundamental change. Put simply: repression does not cause anxiety; rather, anxiety causes repression. An apprehension of danger triggers anxiety, and anxiety brings into play a defensive move. Freud elaborates the idea that anxiety is a defense against fright and situations of danger. *Actual anxiety* is an automatic, inborn response to an external danger, like a battle or a train accident in my earlier examples; *signal* anxiety is a response that anticipates danger on the basis of past experience; it is learned. Freud does not make clear that, while anxiety can be triggered in a quasi-mechanistic way, its psychological content, both conscious and unconscious, has all the richness that is unique to a creature with our peculiar symbolic capacities.

Freud had earlier thought that the purpose of symptom formation was to gratify unconscious wishes while concealing the gratification from oneself. In his new theory the purpose of symptoms is rather to remove the child from a danger situation. The therapist's question remains: 'What is this painful, symptomatic, behavior getting him?' A part of the answer may be the pursuit of pleasure. But the more relevant answer is likely to be, a retreat from greater pain. The exhibitionist who knows he is going to be caught and punished may not like the hurt of the punishment; it may rather be that unsettling someone is an antidote to feeling impotent and helpless. The masochist may not want the pain itself, but seek it as the only condition under which he can allow himself to experience pleasure.

Freud (1926: 166–7) concludes that anxiety has been shown to be 'the defensive behavior of the ego transfigured in a rational light'. He writes:

Anxiety is . . . on the one hand an expectation of a trauma, and on the other a repetition of it in a mitigated form . . . A danger situation is a recognized, remembered, expected situation of helplessness. Anxiety is the original reaction to helplessness in the trauma and is reproduced later in the danger-situation as a signal for help. The ego, which experienced the trauma passively, now repeats it actively in a weakened version, in the hope of being able itself to direct its course . . . The individual will have made an important advance in his capacity for self-preservation if he can foresee and expect a traumatic situation of this kind which entails helplessness, instead of simply waiting for it to happen. Let us call a situation which contains the determinant for such expectation a *danger-situation*. It is in this situation that the signal of anxiety is given.

Other creatures experience *actual* anxiety. They also experience signal anxiety in that they can be trained to avoid something that is connected with a painful stimulus in the past. But because they do not have the symbolic capacities we do, nor perhaps the associative networks of memory, their learned responses to anxiety are more limited than ours. But for any creature the production of signal anxiety is an advance in that it allows the creature to deal more actively with danger situations, or what seem to be danger situations. In human beings, again because of unconscious mental functioning, and implicit and procedural memory, signal anxiety can also trigger responses that keep the source of the anxiety hidden.

Here is an example of signal anxiety in action. Hal is a man in his earlier twenties with a long history of abandonments, a history that colors his response to criticism. He is chronically alert to it, and ready with defense. Hal spent most of one hour telling me how he just could not make sense of a body of literature on which he was to be tested for a promotion. He complained how hard these texts were, how they were making him feel stupid. Maybe he should return, he mused, to the menial work he had had before moving to this new job.

As the hour went on, I became frustrated because I know the books he was referring to, and I think they are genuinely hard to understand, not because they are deep but because the authors are unclear. I did not say this, because it would not have been appropriate. I said instead that perhaps he did not feel he had the right to be critical of the books his superiors had recommended. I was holding back what I really wanted to say, and I could sense frustration in my voice.

Hal is an astute reader of other people's feelings; so I was wondering if I was going to hear from him about my tone. He began the following hour by saying, 'That was a weird session yesterday.' He said he realized that he had been doing something 'regressive'—his word—hoping I would solve a problem for him that of course only he could solve. He said he seemed to have slipped back into the mode of 'I can't do anything', 'I don't know anything', that we had been talking about for a while. 'Taking on this job has really been frustrating to me, and now I have this big challenge ahead of me. I just have a hard time bearing frustration.' He said he recognized that he was just going to have to grow up and accept the fact that there were many things no one could do for him. He then remarked that after the previous hour he had for the first time in a long while had the urge to quit therapy. The thought probably came, he said, from the fact that I had disappointed his 'childish' wish that I could do everything for him.

I said I was struck by his urge to quit therapy the previous day. I concurred that, as we had seen many times, he often played dumb as a way of avoiding taking on a position of authority, and I wondered if in this instance too that was what he was doing: perhaps his know-nothing stance was now, also, a way of avoiding something more painful. I wondered aloud if maybe this urge to quit had to do with something I had done that upset him.

He continued to talk about how it was all just his problem, about how he was asking too much from me, and so on. Then he remarked that he had felt my frustration during that hour. He said that his father had always been exasperated and frustrated with him, and he reminded me of a few incidents that we had talked about a number of times. He said again that he had thought I must have been frustrated in the preceding hour.

I believed that Hal was now occupied with the past in order to avoid anxieties about the present. I said:

'What did you think I was frustrated about?'

'Well, the way I seemed to be regressing and spinning off.'

I said I did not feel we had yet put our finger on what had happened between us that made him want to get out of therapy. It must have been something pretty alarming. But he persisted with his self-accusations.

After some hesitation I said, 'I think I should tell you that I *was* feeling frustrated. Not with you. I felt you were giving those texts too much power. Why that should have frustrated me is my problem. But the point is that you picked up on my feeling, which you then interpreted in your own way. We need to understand what felt so awful that you thought of quitting.'

Hal began associating to incidents in which he had been so furious with a lover or a friend that he had just walked out on them.

'What made you furious?'

After a while he said, 'I was scared. You know my friend Amy? I thought she was going to leave me.'

'So then were you perhaps afraid when you heard my frustration that I would leave you?' He was quiet for a minute, and then he said, 'I think so.'

I said it seemed to me that, with me in the earlier hour, and with Amy, and in all the other episodes he had just been telling me about, he was responding to something the other person really was doing or feeling that made him so anxious that he leaped over the anxiety into his chronic self-recrimination. I suggested that it protected him from acknowledging the importance to him of the real relationship, and therefore from anxieties about loss. He replied, 'It happens in a nano-second.' The 'it' referred to the mental jump he had made from what I infer was a barely conscious hint of anxiety to habits of attention that lead him in another direction.

The way signal anxiety had been working for Hal prevented him from acknowledging how much he values his important relationships. It rendered him unable to do what he can to secure them, even put him in the unwitting position of sabotaging them. And it confused him about whom it is he is now afraid of losing.

Pavlov and Freud both understood that anxiety and fear can be learned; both viewed signal anxiety as adaptive in function. But Pavlov's theory requires no positing of specifically mental states like belief and desire. Freud's explanations of behavior, on the other hand, always include, and necessarily so, reference to how the creature— human child or adult—interprets what happens to him or her; and also takes into account how we deal with the minds of others. The dangers feared by a child are intersubjective in that they refer to beliefs about the mental states of others, the fear, for example, of the loss of love. Freud's theory alone takes into account two obvious yet portentous facts. The first is that the human infant is dependent on those who care for him far longer than are the young of any other species; the second is that in this long period the human infant is developing capacities for symbol formation that are unique to him and that inflect his experiences. In human beings love is then both more important in development and more plastic than it is in other animals.

Freud knew early on how memory can lapse, reinterpret, associatively link one experience to another in thoroughly idiosyncratic ways. He also knew that, because he has language, the human child is able both to see the world under multiple descriptions—his father *as* a fireman, *as* the boss of his friend's father, *as* threatening to leave the mother, *as* falling short of the child's ideals—and to form an inner world of beliefs, desires, fantasies, emotions, and so on, as creatures who lack our cognitive capacities are not. Because of language we are meaning-minded; because of the complexity of our language, because of our skill for *seeing as,* and our memory systems, both the real and the imagined dangers are multiplied. For us, perceptions of things in the external world are colored by our life histories; and the dangers can themselves be 'inner' in the form of our own wants and beliefs. More various also are ways in which we attempt to regain a sense of control: we fantasize that our powers are far greater than they are; we fasten on things in another that allow us to feel contempt, in defense against acknowledging the shame we feel of ourselves; we become violent.

Ironically, the danger situations can include anxiety itself, since a sufficient degree of it can be overwhelming. In their total dependence on the external world for moment-to-moment survival, children need to be biologically equipped to defend themselves against overwhelming anxiety. Adults who have not outlived their earlier habits of defense may mis-assess both the dangers and their own vulnerability. They may find anxiety so intolerable that they disconnect the signal that alerts them to danger.

The change in Freud's theory of anxiety has profound implications both for the psychoanalytic theory of the mind as a whole and for the theory of practice, though Freud himself did not live to work them out. Wachtel (1993: 39) writes:

Freud had said on a number of occasions that repression was the very 'cornerstone' of psychoanalysis . . . By now identifying anxiety [in Freud (1926)] as the motive underlying repression, Freud had in effect shifted the cornerstone. Anxiety, lying beneath and causing repression should have been the new candidate for the grounding concept . . . The task of therapy, it appears in the light of these new formulations, is not so much to bring to light what the patient has wanted to keep hidden as to help the patient overcome the anxiety that made the hiding feel necessary.

Freud's last theory of anxiety has other implications as well, some of which I have already suggested.

1. The importance of the external world
In 'Inhibitions' Freud (1926: 101–8) briefly recounts the case history of Little Hans and his phobia of horses:

It takes a little time to find one's bearings and to decide which the repressed impulse is, what substitutive symptoms it has found and where the motive for repression lies. 'Little Hans' refused to go out into the street because he was afraid of horses. This was the raw material of the case. Which part of it constituted the symptom? Was it his having the fear? Was it his choice of an object for his fear? Was it his giving up of his freedom of movement? Or was it more than one of these combined? What was the satisfaction which he renounced? And why did he have to renounce it? . . . Here, then, is our unexpected finding: in both cases [Little Hans and the Wolf Man] the motive force of the repression was fear of castration. The ideas contained in their anxiety—being bitten by a horse and being devoured by a wolf—were substitutes by distortion for the idea of being castrated by their father. This was the idea which had undergone repression.

Freud goes on to say that Hans's castration fear is not a manifestation of neurotic anxiety nor is it symptomatic. The symptom consists rather in the 'displacement' of the anxiety onto horses. The anxiety itself is intelligible, given Hans's age and experience. For, suppose he has the idea that women have lost a penis they once had; that he wants physical intimacy with his father as well as with his mother; and that he fears such intimacy requires that, like his mother, he lose his penis. So Hans fears castration as both the precondition and the consequence of gratifying his incestuous desires, in fact even of having them.

The point is not the correctness of Freud's interpretation, but rather that he locates the symptom in a context of reality-oriented beliefs and apprehensions. An instinctual demand, Freud (1926: 126) now says, 'is not dangerous in itself; it only becomes so inasmuch as it entails a real external danger . . . Thus what happens in a phobia in the last resort is merely that one external danger is replaced by another.' That is, the child has various desires that were previously unconflicted; but he comes to fear that the penalty for gratifying them, perhaps even for having them, is something dreadful. A danger that begins as external— say, the possibility of abandonment or loss of love—becomes 'internal' because the child fears that his own desires might cause him to be abandoned.

Psychoanalysis was born, we are used to saying, when Freud gave up 'the seduction hypothesis', the idea that all neuroses are traceable to a real seduction, in favor of the idea that many of the seductions 'remembered' by his patients were merely fantasies. Freud went on to claim that a fantasied seduction can play the same causal role in psychological development as a real seduction, an idea psychoanalysts refer to as 'psychic reality'.

Controversy has swirled around this change for many years. Some critics have scolded Freud for letting the real seducers off the hook (Masson 1984). Others have scolded him for finding seductions where they do not exist (Crews 1995). Many years ago, one of Freud's favorite disciples, Sandor Ferenczi, created a furor with his now famous essay, 'A Confusion of Tongues between Adult and Child,' in which Ferenczi described the way in which the child who has in reality been seduced takes the blame on himself in his need to preserve an image of a powerful and benign, protective figure (Ferenczi 1980). The analyst John Bowlby, interested in the effects of various kinds of real separation, has done some of the most significant research on attachment behavior, for which he was castigated by Anna Freud.[1] She said that Bowlby had turned away from the task of 'psychoanalysis', which is to understand the 'inner' world.

---

[1] One of the most interesting discoveries in neuroscience is mirror neurons, which fire in sympathy when an animal (and presumably an infant) observes the actions of another (Meltzer and Prinz 2002). These neurons constitute a system for the presymbolic acquisition of behaviors and gestures observed in others, providing, it is speculated, a biological base for empathy.

Many of us believe that psychoanalytic theory after Freud, if not Freud himself, took an unfortunate turn in minimizing the importance of the external world, or in not recognizing how inextricable internal and external are from each other. But in 'Inhibitions' Freud has once again given external reality an important place in the formation of symptoms. This, too, is in line with contemporary research, which tells us that reality makes an impact on the mind/brain of the infant before it is able to process it cognitively and before the onset of any defensive distortions (Emde 1983; Stern 1985).

2. The importance of the interpersonal
In his early works Freud had accounted for anxiety in terms of the organism alone, independent of its relations with other people and the external world. He thought, for example, that castration fantasies were hereditary. But he was increasingly impressed by the importance of the child's love relationships in the very structuring of the mind. Trauma came to refer to something specifically interpersonal—for example, the loss of a parent, or an overwhelming fear of such loss (perhaps for a child who has only one parent to begin with). It might include an ongoing, painful childhood relationship, or conflicts that seem to the child seriously to threaten that relationship. It may be traumatic, for example, for a child to grow up with a mother who makes it clear that he has never been wanted, or to be chronically humiliated.

In 'Inhibitions' Freud says explicitly that the earliest anxieties all have to do with separation from the mother, and that these anxieties are thematic for later development. Among the chief traumatic experiences for the human infant are abandonment, whether in the form of actual loss or the loss of approval and love; or guilt for actual or imagined harm one has inflicted on those one loves and on whom one is dependent; or shame and humiliation, again connected with abandonment, as when one unconsciously believes one has been abandoned because of some disgraceful act or defect. Anxiety is a response to experiences or expectations of experiences of separation, loss, and death.

3. Reinterpreting 'libido'
Freud and psychoanalysts after him still find conflicts around infantile wishes that are sexual in a broad sense of the word and around aggression.

But, at least as often, and mixed with these, are conflicts between a need for closeness and the safety it seems to bring, on the one hand, and the urge, on the other, to be an independent agent. In a reinterpretation of the basic biological conflict between the forces of life, *Eros*, and the forces of death, represented by aggression, that Freud posited in 'Beyond the Pleasure Principle', Norman O. Brown (1959) convincingly argues that the conflict is instead within the forces of life, between the wish to regress to an infantile state of symbiotic union, and the progressive need to become one's own person. Unsolved, the conflict leads to a continuing dialectic between the desire for intimacy that spurs withdrawal, and a wish to reject intimacy that returns the person in fear and guilt to the sort of dependence that frightened him in the first place.

4. Symptoms, character, and therapy

Freud's thinking about anxiety was always guided by the idea that the origin of a symptom lies in particular conflicts that are somehow stored in memory. Symptoms were thought to be bits of behavior with specific causes. Bring the repressed memory to light and the symptom will fade away. 'Inhibitions' does not spell out but is working towards, I think, a different idea according to which a symptom is a way of thinking and behaving, initially defensive in function, which over time generalizes to form a feature of character structure. There is childhood conflict, and a defensive way of dealing with it; then the conflict is carried over into a disposition like timidity, or contempt, or a harsh moralism. This attitude in turn will determine what presents itself to the child as a danger; it forms what we might call a framing, attitude. A timid person will feel things to be risky that a bolder person will not; a rigidly moralistic person will see certain actions as disgraceful that another would condone. Defenses then have to be mounted against these new dangers, which may share little content with the original ones.
    David Shapiro (2000: 8) writes:

The mind is not only a coherent organization; it is also, an organizer. Our subjective life is organized by attitudes and ways of thinking that are characteristic of each of us. These characteristics function, also, as a regulatory system. They automatically, reflexively, limit or correct perceptions or reactions . . . that might threaten the individual's stability or a present adaptation, even if that stability or adaptation is a pathological one. A guarded person, say, who is tempted to relax his guard, is likely to notice something suspect in time to annul that temptation. It is the attitude of guardedness itself that translated the sensation of the incipient relaxation into an experience of vulnerability and thereby triggers a corrective reassertion or alertness.

All of us see the world against a certain background of assumptions and experiences. It is the rigidity of neurotic framings that make them neurotic. Again Shapiro (2000: 75):

The restriction of motivational experience implies a restriction, also, of objective consideration of the external situation or figure of interest. A selective picture is constructed in support of what the rigid person thinks he should do, a picture that omits all account for his actual feelings, his wish, and often his action. It omits the actual attractions of the disapproved relationship, the relief offered by drinking, the unpleasant realities of the contemplated move.

In anxiety that misfires, attention is constricted, and desires are constrained in ways that counter the agent's ability to know what he wants and to appraise the world fairly realistically as to how best to satisfy them. Often what is inhibited is the person's sense of his own agency, not just indirectly, but directly, because agency is what makes him anxious: in knowing that I am making a decision, I face the fact that I might make a mistake; that I am not perfect; that I cannot see and control the future; that I am closing off some possibilities; that I risk losing out.

One can attempt to avoid such acknowledgments by disowning agency itself. We are familiar with the ways. I postpone making a decision for so long that eventually it is taken out of my hands. Or I interpret another's remarks about option *a* versus option *b* as telling me that I *ought* to do *a*, or that I *would* do *a* if I were a 'good' person or a 'good' patient, a loving daughter, or a grateful friend; and then I 'obediently' take this as a command that exerts a force upon me from outside. Or I back into a decision, making one small step after another, until finally there is enough momentum to carry me across the line; then I can feel, even with some truth, that I did not really make the decision. Or I say, 'I'm doing this because my mother made me into such a timid person', or 'I just can't help it', or 'My feelings overcame me'.

On Shapiro's view (2000: 25), some pathogenic experience of anxiety in childhood, whether due to real trauma or to imagined expectations of dangers, changes not only the child's memories but also his character. The change may consist in his developing attitudes that are inhibitory, such as a rigid sense of duty, or, if self-assertion and success make him anxious, a propensity toward self-belittlement. Once such a development is underway, the child is no longer the same:

Before, he was only a frightened child; now he has become a passively obedient or timid child. Before, he was frightened of a particular real or imagined danger, and he may well continue to feel threatened by what consciously or unconsciously revived that particular danger. But now, as a timid or passively obedient child, he is threatened by much more than that particular danger or any reminders of it. The nature of what is threatening to the child now is no longer determined only by particular memories or fantasies, but by his present attitudes or personality, by what he has become. If he has become timid, an inconsequential initiative will now feel audacious; if he has become carefully obedient, a trivial infraction will seem grave to him.

Neurotic framings are similar to what Weiss and Sampson (1986) call 'pathogenic beliefs'. Picking up on the idea in 'Inhibitions' that 'the most distinguishing characteristic of the neurotic is the unconscious belief in childhood danger situations', Weiss and Sampson define pathogenic beliefs as distressing constructions of reality, usually unconscious, that link frightening outcomes to normal developmental pursuits. Derived from past painful and typically repressed experiences, these dire beliefs represent major organizing principles of experience. The belief explains something traumatic—always of an interpersonal nature—that the child experienced by saying, implicitly, something like: 'I must be bad; I made that bad thing happen'; or 'If I leave my mother (perhaps by having my own life), she will die'; or 'I am guilty for being the only one to have survived the disaster; I must not succeed in the goals I have set myself' (Gassner 2001).

As organizing principles, the beliefs can have lasting and devastating consequences. A belief is pathogenic not only because it inhibits the pursuit of normal goals, like succeeding at a job you want, or sustaining a close relationship; but also because it closes off perception of the very things you need to notice if you are to achieve your goals, such as what the world is like as it pertains to them, and what you really want. It undermines, not only the sense of agency, but also agency itself.

If a symptom is thought of not as a stereotyped bit of behavior resulting from the interaction of mindless forces within the personality, but as part of a meaningful, originally defensive style of thinking and behaving that has generalized over time to form a feature of character structure, the task of therapy looks quite different: no sudden 'cures' with merely quantitative shifts in underlying dynamics, but the modification of conscious and unconscious pathogenic beliefs and attitudes. The aim of psychoanalysis now is to change character. And, if those neurotic framings that help form character are constructed through anxious imagining, then how anxiety is managed must be a central focus of the therapy.

Do the old anxieties disappear altogether? Probably not. An analyst friend told me of how phobic she had been before her own analysis long ago. Since she was a woman who flew her own plane, drove a tractor, and seemed generally intrepid, I was surprised.

'What were you phobic about?'

She laughed. 'Well, for one, spiders. And we lived in the country. The house was loaded with them. All kinds—smooth, hairy, small, huge. I spent a lot of my childhood doing what I could to avoid them. I still dream occasionally that there's a little spider in a far-off corner, sort of glowing. But they've shrunk.'

3

Keeping Time: Remembering, Repeating, and Working Through

Man learns the concept of the past by remembering.

(Ludwig Wittgenstein, *Philosophical Investigations*)

It is time to rescue the phenomenon of memory from being regarded merely as a psychological faculty and to see it as an essential element of the finite historical being of a person.

(Hans-Georg Gadamer, *Truth and Method*)

In the autumn of 1997, the German author G. W. Sebald gave a series of public lectures in his country on contemporary German literature. His theme was how massively his countrymen had repressed their memories of devastation in the Second World War, and the effects of this repression on their culture. About the response to his lectures Sebald (2003: pp. VII–IX) writes:

much of it was rather bizarre in character. However, the inadequate and inhibited nature of the letters and other writings sent to me showed, in itself, that the sense of unparalleled national humiliation felt by millions in the last years of the war had never really found verbal expression, and that those directly affected by the experience neither shared it with each other nor passed it on to the next generation ... It seems to me that we Germans today are a nation strikingly blind to history and lacking in tradition ... And when we turn to take a retrospective view, particularly of the years 1930 to 1950, we are always looking and looking away at the same time. As a result, the works produced by German authors after the war are often marked by a half-consciousness or false consciousness designed to consolidate the extremely precarious position of those writers in a society that was morally almost entirely discredited.

'Looking and looking away at the same time.' The entire passage is a wonderful telling of some of Freud's major themes.

From some growing concerns about the reliability of memory, Freud was led to the view that temporality is constitutive of the mind, and that the mind can be split along faults that are temporal in character. It is trivially true that the present emerge from the past; Freud's insight was that the present mind contains the past, though often in unrecognizable form. The healing process he calls *remembering, repeating, and working through*. Remembering, unlike its avoidance, repetition, allows for working through: clarifying, and integrating into the fabric of the mind, something previously warded off. The concepts of repression, remembering, repetition, working through, transference, and mourning together draw a conceptual map that Freud continually refined. The patient must come to know not so much that this or that event did or did not happen precisely as he thinks it did, but that it *happened*.

Freud and Breuer took their early ideas about remembering, and remembering as catharsis, from Janet, who viewed memory as the central organizing apparatus of the human mind. Janet's work with hysterics had led him to think that memory can follow two different paths: along one it functions in an automatic way, as it does in other species; along the other, it functions in a narrative way peculiar to us. The distinction corresponds roughly to that made earlier between implicit and narrative memory.

In this narrative way, new experiences are integrated into existing mental schema. With experience of a familiar sort, integration happens naturally and without conscious effort. But experiences that are not merely unfamiliar but also frightening and bizarre may at once have an intense psychic impact, yet be unintelligible. Later such unintegrated experiences may surface as isolated memories, disconnected from the person's sense of her own history. Or they persevere as a kind of a historical hallucination, as they do for holocaust survivors (Laub 1993). Or they are 'remembered' in a displaced, emotionally isolated, trivialized form. Or they are expressed as repetitive, behavioral enactments. In the course of treatment, what had been a traumatic memory becomes a narrative, a story now told, and with all the appropriate feeling, to another person.

Janet (1919–25: 663) writes:

It is only for convenience that we speak of it as a 'traumatic memory'. The subject is often incapable of making the necessary narrative which we call memory regarding the event; and yet he remains confronted by a difficult situation in which he has not been able to play a satisfactory part, one to which his adaptation had been imperfect, so that he continues to make efforts at adaptation.

From his early allegiance to Janet, Freud slowly developed what we now know as the 'Freudian' view of memory. Let me briefly trace that development. In *Studies on Hysteria*, Freud and Breuer echoed Janet's idea in the famous slogan 'Hysterics suffer mainly from reminiscences' (Freud 1893–5: 7). Freud suggests that the splitting-off of psychical groups may be a product of what he calls 'defence'. He agrees that trauma disrupts memory; but, in contrast to Janet's more mechanistic idea, Freud is suggesting, like Sebald, that there is an active avoidance of remembering.

Then in a paper entitled 'The Aetiology of Hysteria' Freud (1896: 192–3) writes: 'the symptoms of hysteria . . . are determined by certain experiences of the patient's which have operated in a traumatic fashion and which are being reproduced in his psychical life in the form of mnemic symbols.' It was in this paper that Freud presented to a scandalized audience 'the seduction theory', that 'at the bottom of every case of hysteria there are one or more occurrences of premature sexual experience, occurrences which belong to the earliest period of childhood (1896: 203). Had he heeded Janet's admonition that 'traumatic remembering' is not truly remembering, Freud might have clarified his thesis by adding that the hysteric's reminiscences are not memories as we ordinarily think of them, that what she suffers from is really a peculiar failure of remembering. Nor is that failure either a true forgetting or a motivated 'forgetting'. Hysterical reminiscence is a state in between remembering and forgetting, in between knowing and never having known.

In fact Freud did soon change his mind about the veracity of memory. Whereas earlier he had taken the patient's account of seduction at face value, concluding that it is memories of real events in the public world that get repressed, he came to think that 'psychic reality', the patient's fantasies about what had happened, is the crucial issue. He wrote to Fliess: 'the psychical structures which, in hysteria, are affected by repression are not in reality memories . . . but impulses' (Freud 1897: 247). Sex keeps its importance in Freud's new view; but the traumatic seductions may have happened only in the patient's mind in the form of conflicted, wish-fulfilling fantasies. Freud's basic point, that one's own idiosyncratic interpretation of reality must figure in any *psychological* explanation of her thought and behavior, is right. Both psychology and philosophy of mind owe Freud a debt for tracing out the complex relationships between world and thought, showing us the various ways in which thought is shaped by conflict, anxiety, and desire. But one can have this point and the world as well.

Philosophical theorists of memory have long been concerned with whether remembering always takes the form of having a mental image. Freud did not ask this question explicitly, but there is an interesting suggestion of an answer in the following passage from 'The Aetiology of Hysteria':

As we know from Breuer, hysterical symptoms can be resolved if, starting from them, we are able to find the path back to the memory of a traumatic experience. If the memory which we have uncovered does not answer our expectations, it may be that we ought to pursue the same path a little further; perhaps behind the first traumatic scene there may be concealed the memory of a second . . . so that the scene that was first discovered has only the significance of a connecting link in the chain of associations . . . it always has more than two links; and the traumatic scenes do not form a simple row, like a string of pearls, but ramify and are interconnected like genealogical trees, so that in any new experience two or more earlier ones come into operation as memories. (Freud 1896: 95–6).

The suggestion is that remembering invokes a vast network of affectively colored beliefs and desires, and that this network forms part of the content of what we call 'a memory'. Freud is beginning to tell us more about what memory in the narrative sense is, and how the transition from trauma to narrative can be made. Remembering is an activity of linking. So forgetting, or not knowing, is often a matter of not linking, or unlinking, or not putting memories that are in fact thematically and affectively related together into a coherent story. To explain these acts of dissolution and isolation, Freud was eventually moved to introduce the concepts of unconscious anxiety, defense, and repression, concepts that began to shape what we know as the specifically 'Freudian' view of memory.

Freud's reflections on remembering deepened next with the idea of 'screen memory', a vivid but apparently trivial childhood memory behind which other important experiences are hidden, and which has been inflected by experiences (and unconscious fantasies) subsequent to the event that memory reports:

The recognition of this fact [that the falsified memory is the one of which we first become aware] must diminish the distinction we have drawn between screen memories and other memories derived from our childhood. It may indeed be questioned whether we have any memories at all *from* our childhood: memories *relating* to our childhood may be all we possess. Our childhood memories show us the earliest years not as they were but as they appeared at the later periods when the memories were aroused. In these periods of arousal, the childhood memories did not, as people are accustomed to say, *emerge*; they were *formed* at that time. And a number of motives, with no concern for historical accuracy, had a part in forming them, as well as in the selection of the memories themselves. (Freud 1899: 322).

The concept of a screen memory, *Deckerinnerung*, is related to that of *Nachträglichkeit*, the idea (later posited in the Wolf Man case) that the mind interprets the past in terms of the present, or in terms of events that happened later than the event itself. In 'A Note upon the Mystic Writing Pad' Freud (1924) described memory as a system for receiving perceptions. But *Nachträglichkeit* shows memory differently: memory is not the passive writing pad but the active writer, assembling, organizing, interpreting, and misinterpreting. In Loewald's words (1976: 299): 'Memory is the action by which some sort of order and organization, some sort of permanence as well as of movement and change, come into the world.'

Nachträglichkeit gave Freud a way of understanding many childhood traumas: because of meanings with which the child has later invested it, an event may become disturbing only after the fact. For example, observing parental intercourse at the age of a year-and-a half might not cause the child anxiety at the time; but if he later comes to believe that women have been castrated, the wish to take his mother's place with his father may carry with it the fearful idea of castration (Freud 1914).

The idea of screen memories has more than this to tell us, however. Since all endeavor, and all interpretation of experience, are governed, on Freud's view, by considerations of pleasure, pain, and defense against anxiety, so too is memory. Memories are layered, and the layering is constrained not only by their temporal but also by their dynamic, or defensive, relations to each other. This that I do remember, painful though it may be, is less painful than that which I have 'forgotten', and will not remember. My guilt for having harmed you may include an unconscious belief that I am omnipotent, which may cover a belief in my worthlessness. One memory can screen, or hide, another from view.

In 'Remembering, Repeating, and Working Through', Freud (1914: 148) remarks on the simple form that remembering took in hypnotic treatment: 'the patient put himself back in to an earlier situation, which he seemed never to confuse with the present one, and gave an account of the mental processes belonging to it.' In therapy as Freud comes to practice it, however, the patient does seem to make this confusion between past and present, much as Janet's traumatized patients also did. The patient repeats past traumas, 'finding' herself again and again in a self-destructive relationship with a man, or sabotaging herself at work, or enacting sexual rituals in which she is master, or slave, or both.

But Freud has broadened Janet's notion of psychic trauma to include any interpersonal situation, often habitual, that evokes intense and unresolved intra-psychic conflict, conflict such that, below the threshold of conscious awareness, the very same activity represents, on the one hand, the gratification of a wish, need, or desire, and, on the other, the doing of something in some way dangerous, forbidden, repre- hensible. And Freud has given up hypnosis for what Breuer's patient Anna O. dubbed 'the talking cure', because the phenomenon of resistance has led him to a more complex picture of the mind than the one with which Janet was working.[1]

Freud now sees that even the 'normal' mind harbors psychological constellations that reflect different periods of the person's development, and that the result is a muddle of past and present that it is the task of therapy to resolve. Freud (1914: 150) writes:

the patient does not *remember* anything of what he has forgotten and repressed, but *acts* it out. He reproduces it not as a memory but as an action; he *repeats* it, without of course knowing that he is repeating it. For instance, the patient does not say that he remembers that he used to be defiant and

---

[1] Many analysts now are uncomfortable with the concept of resistance. Schafer (1982) thinks it unfortunately suggests an adversarial relationship between analyst and patient. Weiss (1986) believes that the patient is unconsciously motivated to disconfirm his neurotic beliefs, not to hang on to them. Both analysts would of course agree that the mind constructs defenses against pain. They are therefore distinguishing resistance from defense.

critical towards his parents' authority; instead, he behaves in that way to the doctor. He does not remember how he came to a helpless and hopeless deadlock in his infantile researches; but he produces a mass of confusing dreams and associations, complains that he cannot succeed in anything and asserts that he is fated never to carry through what he undertakes. He does not remember having been intensely ashamed of certain sexual activities and afraid of their being found out; but he makes it clear that he is ashamed of the treatment on which he is now embarked and tries to keep it secret from everybody. And so on . . . As long as the patient is in the treatment he cannot escape from this compulsion to repeat; and in the end we understand that this is his way of remembering.

Freud calls it 'the repetition compulsion', and 'Beyond the Pleasure Principle' is his attempt to explain it.

Early in this essay Freud (1920: 12) describes anxiety as 'a particular state of experiencing the danger or preparing for it, even though it may be an unknown one'. He goes on to note that veterans, apparently 'fixated' to their trauma, often dream repetitively of just the traumatic events themselves. But this fact does not square with either his view of dreams as attempts to gratify unconscious wishes, or the pleasure principle. He is puzzled. He goes on to describe another repetitive sort of activity, children's play, telling us the now famous story about his grandson:

At the age of one and a half [the child] could say only a few comprehensible words; he could also make use of a number of sounds which expressed a meaning intelligible to those around him . . . He was greatly attached to his mother . . . This good little boy . . . had an occasional disturbing habit of taking any small objects he could get hold of and throwing them away from him into a corner . . . so that hunting for his toys and picking them up was often quite a business. As he did this he gave vent to a loud, long drawn-out 'o-o-o-o', accompanied by an expression of interest and satisfaction. His mother and the present writer were agreed in thinking that this was not a mere interjection but represented the German word *fort* ['gone'] . . . The child had a wooden reel with a piece of string tied around it . . . What he did was to hold the reel by the string and very skillfully throw it over the edge of his curtained cot, so that it disappeared into it, at the same time uttering his expressive 'o-o-o-o'. He then pulled the reel out of the cot again and hailed it by its reappearance with a joyful *da* ['there'] This, then, was the complete game—disappearance and return. As a rule one only witnessed its first act, which was repeated untiringly as a game in itself, though there is no doubt that the greater pleasure was attached to the second act. (Freud 1920: 14–15)

Freud suggests that the game is related to 'the child's great cultural achievement' of allowing his mother to go away without protesting. 'He compensated himself for this, as it were, by himself staging the disappearance and return of the objects within his reach' (1920: 15). Freud offers other possible explanations as well: the child is rehearsing the anxiety caused by his mother's occasional departures, and attempting to master it by taking an active role (the child who plays doctor after a painful visit in which he was himself the patient is a homely example of what Freud has in mind); the child is symbolically making his mother come back; or he is vengefully throwing her away as he feels he has been thrown away.

These explanations are all perfectly compatible with the pleasure principle: the child repeats the unpleasant experience in play only as a necessary prelude to pleasure of an indirect sort—the sense of mastery, or the pleasure of revenge itself. 'The pleasure principle' is a complex concept in that it includes the capacity to sustain unpleasure by taking reality into account and expending energy, as a sometimes necessary if painful route to pleasure. It alludes to a finely tuned system of self-regulation that manages pain, pleasure, the perception of reality, and the avoidance, through an experience of anxiety, of anything perceived as a danger.

But there is another sort of repetition with which the analyst in particular is familiar that stretches the pleasure principle, Freud thinks, beyond recognition: transference. He writes:

Patients repeat all of these unwanted situations and painful emotions in the transference and revive them with the greatest ingenuity . . . they contrive once more to feel themselves scorned, to oblige the physician to speak severely to them and treat them coldly; they discover appropriate objects for their jealousy; instead of the passionately desired baby of their childhood, they produce a plan or a promise of some grand present—which turns out as a rule to be no less unreal. None of these things can have produced pleasure in the past, and it might be supposed that they would cause less unpleasure to-day if they emerged as memories or dreams instead of taking the form of fresh experiences. They are of course the activities of instincts intended to lead to satisfaction; but no lesson has been learnt from the old experiences of these activities having led instead only to unpleasure. In spite of that, they are repeated, under pressure of a compulsion. (Freud 1920: 21).

Thus Freud is led to speculate about an instinct inherent in all living processes that works 'beyond' the pleasure principle. Now instead of a polarity between the instincts of self-preservation and the preservation of the species (sex), he pits Life, Eros—both self-preservation and sex—against death, Thanatos, or the forces of destruction. As a good biologist Freud had to add that of course the death instinct is never visible in its pure state; that, Eros would not permit. But the instinct reveals itself, Freud thinks, in human behavior that is repetitive, regressive, disorganized, and typically destructive. At the elemental level of biology, the death instinct it is an urge to go backwards, to return to a state of absolute quiescence.

Most analysts rejected the idea of the death instinct even at the time. It is, I believe, one of Freud's truly bad ideas. Many of us think that all the phenomena he was trying to understand are better explained, furthermore, by concepts he himself had introduced. I return to these presently. But as a beginning we can recall how tricky anxiety is: an affect whose biological function is to alert us to danger, but that can go wrong in a multitude of ways. In a work later than *Inhibitions*, Freud writes:

Either the generation of anxiety—the repetition of the old traumatic experience—is limited to a signal, in which case the remainder of the reaction can adapt itself to the new situation and proceed to flight or defence; or the old situation can retain the upper hand and the total reaction may consist in no more than a generation of anxiety, in which case the affective state becomes paralyzing... (Freud 1933: 82)

That is, anxiety may fail in its function as signal, reproducing the trauma instead. And indeed anxiety *is* 'beyond' the pleasure principle in the sense that, until one has mastered trauma, he is not in a position to go for pleasure. Anxiety is not merely one painful affect among others, but the expression of a primal need for safety.

A child can flourish only in an environment that is, to echo Winnicott, 'safe enough'. Winnicott's 'good enough mother' neatly condenses the ideas that there is no such thing as a perfect nurturer, with the idea that perfection is not what the child needs. He needs only one who is sufficiently protective, loving, strong, self-confident and content herself, to allow the child to feel recognized as a distinct and separate person who can safely explore the world, trusting that his mother, too, will be safe and will not disappear in his absence. Such a mother must also have the good judgment to know when she can encourage the child to do things on his own, and when, on the contrary, his adventures are perilous. The need for safety is 'beyond' the pleasure principle in that the child will be able to pursue pleasure, to develop his own interests and talents, only to the extent that he can trust his caretakers, and, through them, the world and himself. Hence Erik Erikson called 'Basic Trust' versus 'Basic Distrust' the first developmental stage, affecting all the others through which the child will pass.

In a famous essay in which he draws on Lacan's idea of 'le stade du miroir', Winnicott (1971: 112) asks:

What does the baby see when he or she looks at the mother's face? I am suggesting that, ordinarily, what the baby sees is himself or herself. In other words the mother is looking at the baby and *what she looks like is related to what she sees there.* All this is too easily taken for granted. I am asking that this which is naturally done well by mothers who are caring for their babies shall not be taken for granted. I can make my point by going straight over to the case of the baby whose mother reflects her own mood or, worse still, the rigidity of her own defences. In such a case what does the baby see?

Winnicott's answer is that in such a case the mother's face is not a mirror, that the baby's creative capacity begins to atrophy. What could have been the 'beginning of a significant exchange with the world' is blocked.

But have we answered Freud's question about 'the repetition compulsion'? How do we explain such painfully repetitive phenomena as the man who repeatedly 'finds' himself involved with the same sort of contemptuous and belittling woman? The woman who manages to shoot herself in the foot every time she is on the brink of success? The graduate student who seeks out advisors who remind her of her critical, self-absorbed mother?

Of course every situation, every object, is a repetition in something like the sense that the old philosophic problem of 'The One and the Many' formalizes. Nothing can be recognized, or in that sense known, unless it is assimilated to a familiar pattern: repetition is necessary for learning and for moving forward. This is repetition in its inevitable and beneficent form. It is malevolent when, through anxiety, assimilation of the now present and particular to the familiar past blunts appreciation of the present in all its particularity.

We might translate Freud's question about repetition this way: How can we use the past so that, rather than obscuring the present, it helps us notice what is peculiar about this object or situation in the present? And what is the sort of past that makes this difficult? We need to mark off neurotic repetition from the non-neurotic repetition that is necessary for growth. So Loewald distinguishes active from passive repetition, the first of which is progressive and aimed at mastery of the repeated phenomena. Repetition of this sort leads to experience that can then become organized in new and creative ways. Passive repetition, on the other hand, tends towards a duplication of the old trauma, with no attempt at mastery (Loewald 1980b). But this brings us no closer to an understanding of neurotic repetition, which is now simply renamed 'passive' repetition.

Perhaps more helpful is a distinction between primal and symbolic repetition. The first, early, traumatic experience is preserved in non-representational, affective states and 'motor recognitions' in which actions are set off by 'familiar sensory experiences'. A piece of behavior that is repetitive in a neurotic sense can be seen as putting one's inner, unverbalized, experiences into behavior (Broughton 1993: 455–7).

Psychoanalysts suggest a number of explanations for neurotic repetition, all of which are compatible with each other, and none of which invokes an innate, destructive instinct.

1. *The quest for love.* All of us learn love in whatever relationships, happy or unhappy, that we had as children. An attachment to painful feelings may come with the wish to remain attached to persons with whom our relationships were peculiarly painful (Valenstein 1923). The man a woman picks up in a bar may, consciously, seem to her as different from her father as possible; yet unconsciously she may see him as an appropriate partner for a relationship that has a number of structural similarities to the earlier one.

2. *The desire to master trauma.* We find people in later life who remind us of the ones we loved and needed as children, and unconsciously attempt to reconstruct that earlier relationship, in our imaginations and in reality, hoping that we can make things come out differently.

3. *The wish to disconfirm a pathogenic belief.* We unconsciously look for, and create, relationships that we can (unconsciously) think of as similar to ones in the past as a way of testing out (unconsciously) whether our pathogenic beliefs are true (Weiss 1993). Will my success alienate or humiliate the person I love, as in childhood I believed was the case? Will my father leave me because I am somehow defective?

4. *The nature of pathogenic beliefs, in conjunction with signal anxiety.* Any basic belief or assumption tends to form a horizon against which reality is perceived. The same is true of pathogenic beliefs, and as such they are apt to be self-confirming. We notice those things that fit our beliefs; but when they set off a signal of anxiety, we also defend ourselves against fully registering our perceptions. Something in the present that the patient may have sought, for one or all the reasons above, reminds her of a past trauma; the earlier anxieties are aroused again; and the old emergency behavior goes into action. The trouble, once again, is that neurotic expectations tend to be self-fulfilling. For example, the patient who has learned that it is dangerous to stand up for himself is apt to act in ways that invite others to take advantage of him (Wachtel 1993).

5. *Unconscious guilt, or guilt that is conscious but misplaced.* One may seek to be punished, not recognizing this as his motive.

6. *The nature of defensive fantasy.* Behavior that would seem to an outsider to be simply painful and self-punitive may feel to the agent, through the work of defensive fantasy, like a triumph (the turning of passive into active). Here is an account of a baroque scenario of this sort:

you will find if you get to talk to an exhibitionist, that his purpose in displaying his genitals is not to seduce a woman into making love with him but rather to shock her. If she is upset—is embarrassed, becomes angry, runs away—and especially if she calls the police, he has, he feels, absolute proof that his genitals are important. When you learn that he is likely to exhibit himself following a humiliation earlier in the day, you will be alert to the hostile components he experiences in his excitement. For him, this sexual act serves as a kind of rape—a forced intrusion (at least that is the way he fantasizes it) into the woman's sensibilities and delicacy. If he cannot believe that he has harmed her, the act has failed for him . . . His idea—his fantasy—of what is going on includes, then, the following features. He has done something hostile to a woman; he has been the active force, not the passive victim as he was earlier in the day when someone humiliated him. He has converted this trauma to a triumph, capped by his success in becoming sexually excited . . . He seems to be running great risks: he may be caught and arrested, his family and job put in jeopardy. But the true danger that perversion is to protect him from—that he is insignificant, unmanly—is not out there on the street but within him and therefore inescapable. It is so fundamental that he is willing to run the lesser risk, that of being caught (Stoller 1979: p. xii).

What is going on? Perhaps the patient is a man who experienced humiliation as a child around experiences that, in his mind, had to do with masculinity. He learned to handle this humiliation by imagining (fantasizing), or doing, something that he could construe both as turning the tables on the other, and proving, in the eyes of both the other and himself, his masculine competence. The aggressive exhibitionism he now enacts is itself sexually exciting, addictively so; but, since the excitement occurs in the context of old, unconscious, intra-psychic conflicts, it circles into the same anxieties that the behavior is meant to allay. Unfortunately, as Wilhelm Reich (1949: 226) says, 'the more [the masochist] tries to get out of his suffering the more he becomes entangled in it'. Neurotic strategies have the sad effect of preserving old conflicts much as they were. The repeater, witlessly, congeals the psychic past; preserves, like a moth in amber, his childhood self.

Outside the psychoanalytic situation neurotic repetition tends to hold the neurotic structures in place; inside, it is the path to change. Transference and repetition are closely allied. In transference the patient interprets or attempts to construct the psychoanalytic relationship as a repetition of an old one in just those ways that aroused anxiety. The differences enter with the fact that in the analytic relationship the other player is alert to what is going on, or so we hope, and unwilling to accept the role the patient assigns her. She is then uniquely in a position to bring what was unconscious, either because it was repressed or because it had never been formulated, into awareness. Analyst and patient can together begin to discover what the old anxieties were, see their intelligibility given his situation then, and what sorts of things arouse them now. At the same time the patient can discover that his feelings are out of tune with the present, and interfering with his grown-up needs and desires.

A man in his thirties, whom I shall call Sidney, begins an analysis because of problems at work. Repeatedly he does not complete projects on time, or somehow fails at them. It becomes apparent in his analysis that every time something happens that he experiences as proof of his competence, or as the analyst's gratifying him, he worries that he may have harmed her. Is she feeling abandoned? Demeaned? Together, patient and analyst begin to link the present to childhood experiences of helplessness in relation to a disabled father, and to a fantasy of omnipotence that came to the child's aid. But a child who manically imagines himself as very powerful can also then believe he is responsible for his father's injury, particularly if he had ever had malevolent wishes. Repeatedly, analyst and patient work over the past, and repeatedly the analyst does not fall apart when the patient is successful. Present, neurotic, opaque, anxiety becomes transparent as it is linked to the past.

Freud reminds us of his earliest clinical work with patients who had 'forgotten' traumatic events, or, rather, who had, by 'repressing' them, replaced them with symptoms of various sorts. About the psychoanalytic technique he and Breuer developed, Freud (1914: 147) writes: 'Remembering and abreacting, with the help of the hypnotic state, were what was at that time aimed at.' When the symptoms were remembered, with the appropriate affect, the symptoms disappeared. To account for this Freud theorized that it was the 'damning-up' of affect that was pathogenic. If the affect can be discharged—the meaning of abreaction or catharsis—the symptoms can go away. Remembering is pictured here as the sudden emergence of a past scene.

But in 'Remembering, Repeating and Working Through', Freud says that 'forgetting impressions, scenes, or experiences nearly always reduces itself to shutting them off. When the patient talks about these "forgotten" things he seldom fails to add "As a matter of fact I've always known it; only I've never thought of it."' In obsessional neurosis in particular, Freud goes on, 'forgetting is mostly restricted to dissolving thought-connections, failing to draw the right conclusion and isolating memories' (1914: 148–9). In an aside that we can now understand in the light of LeDoux, Freud remarks that there is a particular class of experiences 'for which no memory can as a rule be recovered. These are experiences which occurred in very early childhood and were not understood at the time but which were *subsequently* understood and interpreted' (1914: 149). We might now reinterpret catharsis as the affective component of implicit memory that, through the analytic process, can be provided with a narrative context.

Freud (1937: 65) became increasingly skeptical about the possibility of an accurate reconstruction of the patient's psychic life. Many psychoanalysts now share that skepticism. Some are even doubtful that we can make any useful generalizations about childhood development. Yet Freud's real insight about the temporal character of mental life is untouched. Loewald (1980: 52) puts it this way: 'the whole orientation of psychoanalysis as a genetic approach to mental life, as an attempt to understand mental disease in terms of the history of mental development and to cure it by promoting a resumption of this history—using the faculty of remembering as the main tool—points to the importance of time as being somehow the inner fibre of what we call the psychical.'

Linking past and present, *remembering, as distinct from repeating,* is the activity through which all experiences acquire their significance; past, present, and future take their meaning only within this linking (Loewald 1980*a*: 142). At best, the activity is constant, reworking the psychic past, making the present available as similar yet different.

A paradigm of working through is mourning. Freud calls it work, 'the work of mourning'. He turns his attention to mourning for the first time in 'Mourning and Melancholia', in which he regards these two conditions as different ways of dealing with loss (Freud 1917). A mourner is a person who has lost someone (in reality or in fantasy, perhaps a real person, but seen under the description of a certain fantasy) he values greatly, and *knows* that he has. The knowing is affective, and it takes time; for it requires discovering again and again that in all the familiar places where the lost object once was, it is no longer.

Proust, as well, talks about the temporal work of mourning, but also about the multiplicity through time that each of us is. Mourning Albertine's departure, Marcel says:

In order to enter into us, another person must first have assumed the form, have adapted himself to the framework of time; appearing to us only in a succession of momentary flashes, he has never been able to reveal more than one aspect of himself at a time . . . In order to be consoled I would have to forget, not one, but innumerable Albertines. When I had succeeded in bearing the grief of losing this Albertine, I must begin again with another, with a hundred others. (Proust 1981: 487)

Mourning acknowledges, as well as the particular, loved, person, the unrepeatability of time; it is to melancholia as remembering is to repetition. Earlier Freud had said that change comes automatically with remembrance and the lifting of repression; but he came to see knowledge and memory as more complex than he had thought. The nemesis of memory is not forgetting, as we might think, but repeating; insight is less a registering of what is before the mind than a process of mourning; mourning is both exploring a lost continent and saying goodbye.

The melancholic behaves much like the mourner, with the difference that, whereas in mourning the world has become poor and empty, as Freud says, in melancholia one experiences the poverty in oneself. Both the melancholic and the mourner have suffered a loss; but the melancholic's love was highly ambivalent, and furthermore he attempts to deny the loss. He will not or cannot go through the mourner's affective moves. Instead he makes a ghost of the lost object, preserving it in fantasy by repetitively acting out its return (Miss Havisham, perpetually dressed in bridal clothes to commemorate the desired event that never took place); or by transferring its significance onto someone else. Or he takes the lost object inside himself, again in fantasy, with the result that now his anger against the object is turned against himself. (What Freud calls melancholia we would now call depression.) While the one who has mourned is free to find a new and genuinely gratifying love, the melancholic is condemned to a passive repetition.[2]

For Freud as for Ricoeur (1984),[3] 'time is a condition of human understanding,' remembering of the attributes that make us human: agency, freedom, self-knowledge. Pathologies of memory are not isolated sores, but mortal afflictions. Something like this view of time and memory informs Homer's *Odyssey*. Homer begins with his hero hidden away on the island of Calypso, who has offered him immortality if he will forget home and stay with her forever. Resistance is difficult; Odysseus dallies with Calypso for ten long years. But finally he insists

---

[2] Some psychoanalysts think that, at times, acting-out may be the necessary prelude to remembering (Broughton 1993).

[3] Frank Kermode remarks that we seem to be able to perceive duration only when it is organized in a narrative way with a beginning, a middle, and an end. We describe the clock as saying 'tick-tock', thus making a tiny narrative out of the sounds. Kermode (1966) describes an experiment in which subjects who listen to rhythmic structures such as *tick-tock*, repeated identically, can reproduce the intervals within the structure accurately, yet cannot grasp the interval between the structures. Narrative is our imposition on reality, but one we cannot do without.

on completing his voyage and returning home to Helen. Homer then moves us backwards in time to the obstacles on Odysseus' homeward journey: the land of the Lotus-eaters, Circe, and the Sirens, who lure sailors to death with their song, the text of which, we are told, is the Trojan War. Why this, we wonder, when Odysseus has himself so many times told us this very story? Why should remembering be in one case a fitting background for his voyage, and in another something he must resist to complete it?

The answer is that the Sirens' song does not merely recall the past, but immures its hearers in it. Calypso would have Odysseus lose the past altogether; the Sirens would replace remembering with repetition; Circe not only makes men forget, but turns them into swine when they do. To lose one's memory, Homer suggests, is to lose one's humanity, one's mind, as the etymology of 'mind' and 'memory' suggests. Mind and the right sort of remembering are present only in each other's company.

At its best, psychoanalytic therapy is a process in which some of the faults between psychic past and psychic present are healed. In this way one can take better care of time, acknowledging the past as *past*, the present as the moment of self-determination, and the future as what one can neither control or foresee. 'Keep': keep back, retain, detain, hold, hold back, preserve, conserve, tie up, inhibit. But also: keep up with, husband, care for, look after, watch over, mind.

PART II
Self, Reality, Other Selves

4
Triangulation: The Social Character of Thought

The internalization in our experience of the external conversations
of gestures which we carry on with others in the social process is
the essence of thinking.

(George Herbert Mead, *Mind, Self, and Society*)

Hamlet needed no audience for his soliloquies. Crusoe could have
thought about his predicament before he met Friday. Descartes performed his meditations by himself. So it can seem that, as Descartes
held, thinking might always be done in solitude, requiring the existence neither of other persons nor of a real external world. The catch is
'always'. Once one has become a thinker, one needs no one else in
order to go on thinking; but this is not to say that one might have been
a solitary thinker from the beginning. On a view that has come to
dominate contemporary philosophy and psychology, a creature develops the capacity for thinking in a specifically human way only in community with others. I will call this the intersubjectivist position.

One of the first thinkers in Anglo-American philosophy to formulate
such a position was George Herbert Mead, who, influenced by Darwin,
attempted to give a naturalistic account of specifically human thought by
tracing it to lower, simpler orders of communication (Mead 1934). At
the same time, Mead insisted that our symbolizing activity is categori-
cally different from any form of communication from which it evolves.

Mead distinguishes three levels of meaning. The first he calls a conversation of gestures, seen among the higher vertebrates. The second is
the signal-language level at which a single word, like 'Fire!', acts as a
stimulus to behavior. Signals should be distinguished from so-called
natural signs: spots as a sign of measles, thunder of rain, footprints of

animal presence. Understanding these as signs requires neither convention nor social interaction. The infant's cry comes closer to communication; yet the infant himself means nothing by his crying. It is a biologically programmed signal of distress. Signals, on the other hand, are social, and they can be learned. (Estrus signals sexual receptiveness, but it is not social in the relevant sense.)

Mead calls the third level *symbolic*. Here is fully articulated propositional thought, in which symbols, which are not context dependent, replace signals that are. By propositional thought I mean thought that links a subject and a predicate, as in asserting or judging *that* something is the case, or regretting *that* it is, hoping *that* it might be, desiring *that* it were. Where one creature understands another's signal only in the context of a common enterprise in which they are engaged (flying north, escaping a predator, looking for honey), this is not so with symbolic communication; I can use and understand the word 'tree' as referring to trees, or the American flag as standing for America, even though there are no trees around; even though we are in Australia. As we might say now, meaning of this sort has *intentionality*: we can communicate *about* something that is not present, calling attention to one of its properties rather than another, so describing the same man as Mary's father, the detective who lives down the block, the murderer of Mary's lover, and so on.

As Grice (1957) later put it, grasping a symbolic communication, whether linguistic or gestural, requires not merely discerning the intention (here 'intention' means aim, or goal) of the other, but also knowing *that* she has an intention, a belief, a goal. When Many says to John, 'Bring me the hammer', Many intends John to understand by these words that she wants him to bring her the hammer. And if her communication succeeds, he knows that this is what she intends him to understand. Not only are *A* and *B* both minded creatures but also, and crucially, each knows that the other is minded like herself. Grice's characterization focuses on linguistic meaning; but it captures as well several features of non-natural meaning, like waving one's hand, drawing on the blackboard, whistling 'Dixie'.

Animals can be trained to use signs that have a conventional meaning—to respond, for example, in a particular way to certain words. They are creatures with aims and goals, intentions in that sense. But we do not have evidence that, for any animal *A*, it understands animal *B* as having intentions whose mental states *A* wants to affect. As Mead puts it, an essential difference between a mere gesture and gesture at the symbolic level is that the latter is accompanied by an 'idea', an idea that is virtually the same for both creatures (I say, 'I am feeling depressed', and, if you catch my meaning, you think, 'She is feeling depressed'.) The question is: how does this phenomenon emerge out of gesture and signal?

Mead answers by positing an identificatory act he calls 'taking the attitude of the other'. The basic idea is that a gesture of the first creature, *A*, takes on a meaning for a second creature, *B*, who responds to *A*'s gesture; in so doing, *B* interprets *A*'s gesture in a certain way. *A* did not intend his gesture to have such a meaning; he did not intend anything at all. Yet, if *A* can now take *B*'s attitude toward his own gesture, he becomes his own interpreter; his gesture acquires for him a meaning like that it has for *B*. I have cast the process Mead envisions as if it takes place in the life of a single individual; but Mead thinks of it as spanning species and generations. At the end of this process, he thinks, a creature with symbolic thought has evolved.

With the ideas of 'internalizing' and 'taking the attitude of the other', Mead hoped to have located a particular bit of behavior that would explain the rise of symbolic thought, while preserving his insight that it is irreducible to anything less complex. The problem with Mead's account, however, is that either *A*'s taking the attitude of the other just is the very thing to be explained, an act of interpretation that presumes symbolic thought; or else there is nothing yet to distinguish what *A* does from mimicry or imitation, and we have not left the conversation of gesture. Of course, if symbolic thinking is not reducible to any set of simpler antecedents, there will in any case be a gap. But perhaps we can go further than Mead did in closing it. Nevertheless, in launching an investigation of meaning from two creatures interacting in a shared world, Mead's argument moves in the right direction. By implication, Descartes's investigation was wrong-headed both because it made the solitary individual its starting point, and because it took reflection rather than purposive, worldly action as the paradigmatic expression of human thought.

During roughly the same period, the Russian psychologist L. S. Vygotsky was developing ideas similar to Mead's. Vygotsky also held that the individual mind emerges from a more rudimentary and collective form of life, and that the crucial turn is a kind of internalization of the other. Critical of Piaget, who held, following Freud, that first there are deeply personal, subjective, autistic mental states, which under the pressure of socialization finally yield to 'social thought', Vygotsky (1962) traced a developmental scheme according to which 'egocentric thought' proceeds to full-fledged mental states. Vygotsky writes: 'the process of internalization is not the *transferral* of an external activity to a preexisting internal plane of consciousness; it is the process in which this internal plane is formed' (quoted in Wertsch 1985: 64). For example, the child reaches unsuccessfully for an object, and the mother comes to get the object for the child. Over time what was at first a gesture that had no significance for the child but only for the mother, becomes, through that interaction, a gesture with which the child *means* to point. By this route, eventually the child as well as the mother can point to the apple with the idea in mind of 'here is an apple'. Daniel Stern's use (1995) of the idea of feedback loops in parent–infant interactions suggests a similar process.

Like Mead and Vygotsky, the later Wittgenstein thought the Cartesian, subjectivist picture fundamentally wrong-headed in isolating thought from action, private thought from public speech, mind from body, one mind from other minds: the idea that individual words or concepts have meaning all by themselves begins its investigation of meaning in the wrong place, for words come to have meaning only through the activities of actual speakers who are doing things with words in the course of carrying out communal enterprises (Wittgenstein 1953). On the Wittgensteinian view, our lives as thinking creatures can be divorced neither from our lives as acting creatures, nor from our engagements with others. We acquire the concepts of belief and desire, but also of apple, mother, love, by engaging in various communal practices, like pointing to an object in the presence of another, or playing games with him, or carrying out or refusing to carry out a request. Children do not learn that oranges exist, that beds exist. They learn to peel oranges, to lie in beds. Attention to the ways language is actually used in daily life will free us from the temptation to hypostatize language and meanings, as Plato did in positing a realm of abstract, immutable, Forms. There are not *meanings*, but people meaning things by what they say and do.

Wittgenstein suggests that the ability to use symbols, to have concepts, requires a kind of rule following, where a rule is by nature something that has its meaning only within a community. By rule following Wittgenstein means something other than the mere disposition to do as others do, for bees and lemmings, and indeed all other creatures, are so disposed, yet we can describe their behavior without ascribing to them concepts. Mere regularity of behavior, even regularity that is social in character, does not give us the rule following Wittgenstein is trying to capture. Nor does discriminatory behavior: sunflowers can turn toward the sun, thermostats register degrees of heat, bulls be enraged by the color red, all in the absence of concepts, symbols, thought.

Wittgenstein must have had in mind, Davidson argues, that the creature must understand that some things are *correctly* included under the concept and some things are not, that some applications of it are right, and some wrong, if we are to attribute concepts to the creature in the first place. How do I sometimes know what I mean? A necessary condition is that I have the ideas of a correct and an incorrect use, since without these ideas there is nothing to give content to the idea that we sometimes *know* what we mean. To know the meaning of a word or a concept is to know how to use it; and no mental item such as an image, or an idea, or a rule, can itself tell us how a word or a concept is to be used. Knowing the use of an expression requires, rather, that one be a member of a community whose life one shares, since only public uses of language can provide the idea that one may be using a word or a phrase correctly or incorrectly. Not that what others say is always right, but that understanding their practices is necessary for acquiring the very ideas of correct and incorrect, right and wrong, true and false, mind, itself.

This makes normativity central to what Mead called symbolic thought; and it brings sentences, even one-word sentences like 'Mama!', to the fore of our investigation. For words are learned in context, and the context is asking for help, or making an exclamation, or affirming, or doubting, or protesting. We are interested not in isolated symbols but in propositional thought, in how the child learns to say it is or it is not so.

What is involved in having belief that is propositional in character, Davidson asks? To believe that *p* is to hold that *p* is true. Of course you can know that it might be false, can be doubtful of its truth, and so on; the point is that the concepts of belief and truth, evidence and reason, are necessarily linked. So, if you have a belief of a propositional sort (the beliefs we may attribute to animals other than ourselves are presumably not propositional in character), you must have a grasp of the distinction between how you *think* things are and how they (truly) are, between right and wrong, correct and incorrect, true and false, since belief is, by definition, a state of mind *about* the world; it is the sort of thing that can be true or false (even though one may never know in a particular case which it is), and for which one adduces evidence and reasons.

The goal, then, is to say what we can about how a child might get hold of the distinctions between the false and the true, between how things *seem*, and how they objectively *are*. As Richard Rorty (1998) writes, 'The key to understanding the relation between minds and bodies is not an understanding of the irreducibility of the intentional to the physical but the understanding of the inescapability of a normative vocabulary. For the inability by an organism to use such a vocabulary entails that the organism is not using language at all.'

To account for normativity we must posit a kind of triangulating process, as Davidson (1989, 1992) calls it, in which child and adult communicate, at first not in words on the child's part, of course, about an object in the physical world they share. Davidson sketches a primitive learning situation. The mother hands the child an apple, saying 'apple' as she does. Mother and child are together interested in the apple, and interested also in each other's response to it. The child babbles, and at some point, in this or a similar exchange, the child hits on a sound close enough to 'apple' so that the mother rewards the child with a laugh, intensified interest, more play, or any of the other kinds of responses that infant observers have described. The mother has in mind the apple when she says 'apple', and apple is what she means by the word. But at what point can we say that 'apple' is what the child herself means? So far, there is nothing to distinguish the mother's response to the child from an observer's response to a trained dog. So our story about the child needs a more complex form of triangulation than the one we have so far described.

What it needs is a very particular sort of interaction between child and mother in which they can observe an object in common, and observe also each other's responses to that common object. The child must be responding to a specific object, and she must know that the mother is responding to that same object. Over time, the child correlates the mother's responses to the object with her own.[1] So the object must be something public, discernible by both mother and child, to which, furthermore, they can give a name that will allow them both to refer to it even in its absence. They must be responding to the same object in the world; they must be responding to it in similar ways; and they must both observe that they are.

In such a situation it will sometimes be the case that mother and child respond to the same thing, something they can both see to be the same thing, differently. The questions can then arise: Who is right, she or I? What is the object really like? What does she see that I don't? Or, What do I see that she doesn't? It is this sort of situation that makes room for the normative concepts of error, right and wrong, true and false, my view of things versus hers, my view versus the way things (objectively) are. Such an interaction not only allows the mother to say of the child, 'She is seeing an x'; it allows the child to say, 'I am seeing an x' (or 'I want an x', or 'I am thinking about an x').

We have been talking about the public aspect of thought; but thought is also subjective and private. While the first concepts the child learns are tied to a public language and a public world, every concept quickly acquires resonances that are unique to the child; so the child is acquiring an idiolect, a way of thinking, that is hers alone. Some of these private thoughts are inarticulate, and unconscious, often because they have not been articulated to another.[2] The important point is that private thought of this sort does not precede communication, but depends upon it.

The interactions I have been discussing *make room* for normativity, Davidson emphasizes; they do not fully explain it; triangulation is a necessary but not a sufficient condition. This is to reiterate that thought is irreducible to any of the prior conditions we can specify, without

---

[1] Winnicott's writings about the transitional object are onto a similar idea. The concept of reality is constructed for any child, Winnicott suggests, through her (triangulating) interactions with some loved external object and a loved other person who is responding both to her and to that same object. Such an object can then become symbolic, say of the breast. Winnicott (1971: 6) writes: 'When symbolism is employed, the infant is already clearly distinguishing between fantasy and fact, between inner objects and external objects, between primary creativity and perception.' Yet, while Winnicott thinks that before this time there are inner objects, I want to say that only when there are, for the child, objects that are truly public can there also be 'objects' that are truly inner in a subjective, inner world.

[2] This is a point with which Davidson might not agree.

covertly including thought itself among those conditions. The search for something more, for necessary *and* sufficient conditions, is tempting: since mind cannot come into being unless all the physical properties and worldly conditions necessary to sustain it are present, one might hope to identify mind with these conditions, or some subset of them.[3] But mind confronts us with what Polanyi (1958), much earlier than contemporary complexity theory, called 'emergent properties', properties that arise spontaneously from elements at preceding levels and that are not specifiable or predictable in terms of them.

Nevertheless, by introducing the ideas, first, of normativity, and, second, of the necessity of a real, shared world, in which a triangulating relationship can take place, we know a little more about the space in which thought arises.

Davidson argues for triangulation on strictly logical and conceptual grounds. But there is a good deal of evidence for it in psychological studies of infant–child engagements. These include predictable formats of interactions (Bruner 1983), and the kind of affect attunement and mutual responsiveness between mother and baby that Stern and Trevarthan write about: pointing to objects, joking together, playing games, taking turns. The essential condition, again, is not merely that infant and caretaker can point to the same object, but that they can observe each other making this reference.

Some psychologists locate particular points along the developmental route, among them 'the nine-month revolution', when, for the first time, infants begin to make attempts to share the attention of an adult, and the understanding of false belief, which takes place much later, around the age of 4 or 5.[4] On the basis of observing parents with children, Fonagy and Target argue that a child's understanding of the mental world, her having 'a theory of mind' (Premack and Premack 2003), is a developmental achievement that requires mutual interaction and recognition. By the age of 3, many pieces of it are in place: the child has thoughts in the form of what Fonagy and Target call first-order

---

[3] Some of the current interest in consciousness seems to be motivated by such a hope: surely there must be, some philosophers, psychoanalysts, and neurologists think, some particular set of neural connections that will explain consciousness so thoroughly that we can say, this *is* consciousness.

[4] Trevarthan (1979); Kaye (1982); Stern (1985, 1995); Wellman (1992); Fonagy (1996*a*, *b*); Tomasello (1999).

representations; she has symbolization, and, in general, the distinctions between playing and reality, dream images and thoughts, on the one hand, and things in the real world, on the other. The child can distinguish between reality and 'psychic reality'; for example, she can pretend that her father is a dragon, yet know he will not breathe fire, and that the same fatherly, familiar figure who is now the dragon will put her to bed. But the distinction between pretend and for-real is not firm; the child cannot easily go back and forth between them, keeping their difference clear. And, because the pretend mode is not yet firmly grasped *as* pretend, it easily becomes psychically 'real', hence frightening. What the child lacks is the capacity for second-order representations, that is, thoughts *about* her own 'representations', her own mind.

By the time she is 4 or 5, Fonagy and Target continue, the child can in the normal case understand both another's behavior in terms of mental states and her own, recognizing in each case that these mental states are representations that are based on one of many possible perspectives, and understanding that they are therefore fallible. In this sense the child now has not only first-order but second-order representations. It is a new step, for which the child needs repeated experience of her own current feelings and thoughts, and the frame that the adult's normally reality-oriented perspective provides (Fonagy 1996*a*). In this account we have once again the idea that the ability to interpret the minds of others goes hand in hand with the understanding of one's own mental states, and vice versa.

I would emphasize an aspect of this triangulating process that Fonagy and Target perhaps take for granted: the 'object' in question is a real person with whom the child is in communication, about a real external world, with material objects in it. So modified, their view is this: the child needs the repeated experience over time of seeing that her own mental attitudes *toward something present to both her and an adult* are recognized by the adult, and of seeing that the adult's attitudes *toward this same thing* are different from the child's. This same thing must be something clearly observable and common to the spatio-temporal world they share. (Later on the 'thing' might be propositional in nature: *that* the earth is round, *that* my mother used to sing to me, *that* psychoanalysis is not a science.) The perception of something that is the same, outside both persons' minds, is necessary for the perception that they are perceiving or thinking of it differently; and those dual perceptions are necessary for the further idea that one of these perceptions may capture something about the object that the other perceptions do not.

It is important to single out propositional thought as the specific form of human thinking for the following reasons. Only thought of a propositional sort has implications, makes assertions, sometimes contradicts itself, commits the thinker to certain conclusions, invites challenge or trust on the part of another, makes promises and reneges on promises, is open to doubt, challenge, question, reflection. Only propositional thought makes a place for dialogue that is both interpersonal and intrapersonal: I can wonder what I mean by what I said, I can ask you what you meant by what you said. Only thinking of this sort can be said to be rational, and also, irrational: self-deceptive, foreclosing reflection, oblivious to the implications of one's thoughts, dissociating one's experiences or beliefs, or not recognizing a fantasy for what it is. It is propositional thought that has clearly departed from the realm of stimulus response.

Our developmental picture now looks like this. From the beginning, infants make sounds and gestures that their caretakers take as signs of the infant's wants and needs. But the infant only gradually becomes able herself to mean something by what she says and does. The implication is not that before the infant has propositional thoughts and intentional states, nothing at all is going on in her head, though it is hard to say what is. At the very least infants have feelings, emotions, sensations, purposes, instincts; they communicate, perceive, and learn. Infant watchers have learned that early infant–parent exchanges have much to do with whether the child begins to feel that she can, or cannot, make herself understood; that she has, or does not have, something valuable to say or to give (a child who is not noticed, not listened to, may come to believe, by way of defending her parent, and herself from anger toward him, that she is not worthy of being understood); that she is more or less at home in the world, or, dangerously omnipotent, at its edge. Infant research is useful in showing how patterns of interaction between infant and caretaker can very early establish habits of response that later might be expressed as core beliefs such as 'I had better not let on that I know what I know', or 'I deserve every bad thing that happens to me', or 'I am [or am not] able to cope with new tasks', or 'the world is a fearful [or an exciting] place'.

The practices of interpreting another, asking him and oneself for evidence and reasons, pointing out that this remark or this judgment is not consistent with others, mark the very space of reasons the child enters, and must enter, in learning how to think. Of course the inter-personal relations that initiate the child into it are not coolly rational but fraught with other lessons about loving and losing, abandoning and being lost, wanting and not having, lessons that can cramp as well as nourish thinking.

There are obvious similarities between the concept of triangulation I am urging and those of a number of psychoanalytic writers. Ronald Britton (1989) (following Bion) writes that the child's acknowledgment of the parents' relationship with each other creates 'a triangular space' in which thinking can occur. Green (1993: 285) writes that Winnicott's 'transitional object' describes not so much 'an object as a space lending itself to the creation of objects'. Ogden (1994: ch. 5) develops a concept of 'the analytic third', according to which 'the analyst gives voice to the experience of the analysand as experienced by the analyst', thus providing, as I think of it, a third perspective from which the analysand can see himself.

My picture of triangulation differs from Britton's and Green's in insisting not only on the presence of real persons besides the child, but also on a real, material world, which they share. This is a developmental thesis; but not only. It is also a claim that the very possibility of dialogue presumes a common frame and common points of reference. The analysts I have just mentioned intuit this idea, I believe, in positing a triangular 'space'. But it has to be made clear that this space and the objects in it are not merely psychological; the frame cannot itself be yet another mental 'representation'. It has to be something steady, something outside both minds.

It is this last idea that presents a challenge to those many psycho-analysts who wish to abandon altogether the idea of reality as some-thing objectively real, the (partial) cause of, but not identical with, our individual experiences. As I say in the Appendix, analysts are lured in an anti-realist direction not only by the arguments of the traditional philosophic skeptic and his newer postmodernist relatives, but also by considerations specific to psychoanalysis. First of all, there are the challenges to the reliability of memory. Then there is the particularly psychoanalytic emphasis on the role of individual history and needs in the forming of perceptions. Finally, there is the contemporary analyst's wish to dissociate herself from what she sees as an authoritarian presumption that her beliefs are more accurate and reliable than the patient's: she wants to acknowledge that she, too, sees the world from her own subjective perspective.

Under the weight of all this, the concept of reality has been disappearing from contemporary psychoanalytic theory. The following passages exemplify this trend.

1. ' "Reality", as we use the term, refers to something subjective, something felt or sensed, rather than to an external realm of being existing independently of the human subject' (Atwood 1992: 26–7).

2. The idea of analytic 'objectivity' is 'an intellectual remnant of the one-person psychology paradigm. . . . Might reducing the object of analysis to the "interaction" between patient and analyst not mislead us, if it predisposes us to imagine that there is an objective reality, "out there" between analyst and patient, that one can be "objective" about' (Fogel et al. 1996: 885).

3. 'The psychoanalytic task is not trying to discover something that was already there, in the patient's mind, but trying to devise a view of [his] life, present and past, that *works*, i.e. that helps him feel better' (Renik 1998: 492).

But how do analyst and patient even get started on the process of understanding each other's particular points of view without triangulating on what they share in common? The danger, of course, for the analyst is that she will presume the particular quality of the patient's attitudes to be more like her own than they are. Both analyst and, eventually, the patient must be willing to abandon any one premise about their common ground. But they cannot abandon them all and still begin to make sense of each other.

Yes, each of us constructs *a picture* of reality. No two pictures are identical. All are open to revision. What keeps pulling us back to the drawing board is the world itself.

5
On Judgment

There are three truths: my truth, your truth, and the truth.

(Peter Brook, *Tierno Bokar*)

We can define thinking so broadly as to include the activity of chimpanzees, parrots, even machines; or more narrowly in a way that perhaps singles out human beings. Freud (1911: 219–21) locates the narrower definition in the following well-known passage:

Instead of (hallucinatory wish-fulfillment), the psychical apparatus had to decide to form a conception of the real circumstances in the external world and to endeavor to make a real alteration in them. A new principle of mental functioning was thus introduced; what was presented in the mind was no longer what was agreeable but what was real, even if it happened to be disagreeable. This setting-up of the *reality principle* proved to be a momentous step . . . The place of repression . . . was taken by an *impartial passing of judgment*, which had to decide whether a given idea was true or false—that is, whether it was in agreement with reality or not.

Let us reflect on the notion of judgment as Freud spells it out in this passage.

In secondary process the mind has to decide, Freud says, whether 'an idea' is true or false. 'Idea' is a notoriously ambiguous term in philosophy, referring variously to sense-data, concepts, beliefs, and propositions. In this passage 'idea' has to mean proposition, since only beliefs and sentences that express propositions can be said to be true or false. Judgment, then, requires the capacity to think in ways that propositions capture.

The ability to make judgments does not demand that all one's thoughts be propositional, only that one be able to entertain propositional thoughts such as 'This table is rectangular', or 'Johnny stole the apple', or 'Mother left home just a few minutes ago', the capacity—put grammatically—to link a subject with a predicate. Judgment is 'the faculty, *not the desire*, of affirming and denying . . . the faculty by which the mind affirms or denies what is true or false', Spinoza (1963: 75; writes emphasis added).

What is implied in the concept of truth? I am not asking how in any instance we know the truth, but what we mean by saying that a belief or sentence is true. What must a creature who has the concept of truth understand? Thought is *about* something; if a proposition is true, things are as it says they are. Thoughts refer, designate, symbolize. Having the concept of truth requires knowing, then, that thought is distinct from what it is about, that a thought is a mental, subjective state about an objective reality. The idea of representation in one of its many senses is what this idea of aboutness captures. It is because thought has this peculiar distance from the world that it can get things wrong, imagine, distort, fantasize, remember things past, envision the future.

In calling 'the setting-up of the *reality principle*' a 'momentous step', Freud is explicitly contrasting judgments about things as they are with wishes, or expressions of personal taste, or sentences that look like judgments about what is but that are really expressions of disguised wishes. With judgment, we might say, come the capacities for reality testing, and also for fantasy, self-deception, delusion, and illusion.

Judgments aim to say how things objectively are, not just how they look to me. Implicitly Freud invokes the idea of something that exists outside my particular experience, my partial perspective, that is in principle available to us all. You and I can both believe there is a unicorn in my garden. We may both be right, or both be wrong; or one of us may be right, and the other wrong. Objective reality is that about which true and false judgments can sometimes, in principle, be made, whether the 'something' in question is material, or mental and itself subjective. We each have beliefs not only about apples and storms, but also about what other persons *believe* and *intend* in relation to this apple and that storm; we love, hate, are angry, forgive, and we have beliefs about such attitudes of our own and of others. (The material world is only a part of objective reality. Mental states are also real in that we have beliefs about them, beliefs that again may be true or false.)

The idea of the 'objectively' real is the idea of there being something that is the focus of agreement and disagreement, about which it is possible to get evidence, to engage in dialogue, to agree and disagree, and sometimes to arrive at a common view. *It is not the common view itself.* The concepts of objective reality, of the true and the false, rest essentially on the distinction between my subjective perspective on things and yours, on the understanding that things look different to you from where you stand from the way they do to me from where I stand. So the idea of perspective is also contained in the idea of judgment.

'Truth' is a word with content only in an interpersonal world; only in such a world can there be 'my' truth, or the world as I subjectively see it; and only if I acknowledge a public world about which things can be objectively true or false is dialogue between us possible. Think of the beliefs of each one of us, said the African sage Tierno Bokar, as a small arc of a circle. If I turn my arc away from yours, insisting that 'my truth' is the only truth there is, I lose sight of the circle. The world itself disappears, and with it the possibility for dialogue between us.

Perspective is a tripartite concept: first, other creatures like myself have minds, with beliefs formed from particular angles on the world; second, the world itself can be seen in different ways, or under different aspects, or, as philosophers say, under different descriptions; third, these points of view are in a very particular sense intersubjective; they can to some extent be shared. I may take your 'point of view' in the literal, spatial, sense, if I come into your garden and see how my garden looks from yours. A similar sharing of mental gardens also happens: I can understand that you have the beliefs you do about a particular event or object, and why you do, even if the beliefs are different from mine.

We sometimes speak of logic as giving 'the laws' of thought. For example, the 'law' of non-contradiction states that x cannot be both a and not-a at the same time and in the same respect. In what sense is this a law? It is certainly not a generalization induced from particular events. Nor is it a convention on which we agree: we do not learn to think and speak and then, from somewhere beyond our activities as thinking, communicating creatures, actively engaged in the world, decide that this is a law we will observe. Rather, the 'law' of non-contradiction formulates a condition of thinking and speaking, of our understanding ourselves and each other. We can see this if we attempt to imagine a creature who chronically asserted—not using the predicates ambiguously, nor joking or making a dramatic point—that something is and is not a square, or red, or a person; such a creature would be unintelligible both to us and to itself. Our lives as thinking, acting beings presume that we are already at home in logic: only thoughtful creatures can see some of thought's essential forms.

On the view just laid out, it is clear that a judgment is not merely a conglomeration of simpler units. Hume had hoped to show that it was. In *The Treatise on Human Nature* he tried to derive judgments from *impressions*, or *sense-data*, and the mental copies of sense-data in the form of what he called *ideas*. He held that the mind is carried from one idea to another along a route of association, such as contiguity in space and time, or causality. But the project did not work. His afterthoughts to the *Treatise* sadly conclude:

there are two principles, which I cannot render consistent; nor is it in my power to renounce either of them, viz. *That all our distinct perceptions are distinct existences, and that the mind never perceives any real connexion among distinct existences.* . . . For my part, I must plead the privilege of a skeptic, and confess, that this difficulty is too hard for my understanding. I pretend not, however, to pronounce it absolutely insuperable. Others, perhaps, or myself, upon more mature reflexions, may discover some hypothesis, that will reconcile these contradictions. (Hume 1951: 636)

In viewing judgment as a capacity that emerges through a developmental process to which bodily need is crucial, Freud took a fundamentally different tack in the right direction. The baby is in want; it comforts itself through an act of imagination, the 'hallucinated breast' in the passage I quoted earlier. But the *pure* pleasure principle cannot survive for long: disappointment forces the infant to take a detour to pleasure rather than a straight shot. First there is the pleasure of a wish fulfilled, then disappointment; first self, then other; first magic, then 'secondary process' thought. With the introduction of the reality principle, Freud (1911: 222) remarks, 'one species of thought activity was split off; it was kept from reality testing . . . This *activity* is *phantasying.*' Freud is setting the stage for an account of neurosis as a later attempt to circumvent pain and external reality by turning to imaginary satisfactions.

Summarizing Freud's theory, Rapaport (1967) says that first there are two qualities, pain and pleasure, in terms of which tension becomes conscious; then hallucinatory wish-fulfillment introduces new conscious qualities that yield thoughts; and, finally, disappointment engenders the thinking of thoughts.

Neither Freud nor Rapaport attempts to spell out the route from thoughts to thinking, nor from the pleasure principle to the 'linking' involved in judgment. Klein and Bion do. They return to Humean building blocks in the form of phantasies.[1] Thinking depends, Bion says, on the successful outcome of two developmental processes, the first of thoughts, the second of 'an apparatus' (Freud's word) to cope with thoughts. Bion (1988: 179) goes on to remark that 'this is different from any theory of thought as a product of thinking, in that thinking is a development forced on the psyche by the pressure of thoughts and not the other way around'.

The infant, Bion claims, has an *a priori* knowledge of the breast. Bion speaks of this knowledge also as an inborn disposition to expect the breast, also as a 'preconception'. When the *preconception* is brought into contact with the realization, there is then a *conception*. At first the infant is not aware of a need, for example, for the breast, because such an awareness would require 'thought', a term Bion (1977: 34) reserves for what he calls the linking of a preconception with a frustration. Converting absence into presence, the infant experiences the aware-ness of the need not satisfied as a bad breast that is present:

as far as I can make out ... the infant is aware of a very bad breast inside it, a breast that is not there and by not being there gives it painful feelings. This object is felt to be 'evacuated' by the respiratory system or by the process of 'swallowing' a satisfactory breast. This breast that is swallowed is indistin-guishable from a 'thought' but the 'thought' is dependent on the existence of an object that is put into its mouth ... The breast, the thing in itself, is indistinguishable from an idea in the mind ... The realization (of the desired object) and the representation of it in the mind have not been differentiated. (Bion 1977: 57–8)[2]

If the capacity to tolerate frustration is sufficient, the 'no-breast' inside becomes a thought, and an apparatus for 'thinking' it develops.

---

[1] British psychoanalysts use the spelling 'phantasy'; Americans use 'fantasy'. The first invokes the specifically Kleinian concept of fantasy that I describe in this chapter.

[2] In his idea of 'the thing in itself', Bion refers to Kant explicitly. But Kant had in mind an order of reality that can never be experienced. This is not how Bion uses the idea in this passage.

Here is another of Bion's pictures. First there are stimuli—he also calls them sense-data—that are colored by frustration, pain, and pleasure. Sense-data precede both conscious and unconscious thought, so, until sense-data are somehow converted into thoughts, thinking cannot take place. This conversion requires that the sense-data be cast in a corporeal form, the process we described a moment ago in which the infant feels a need not satisfied as a bad breast that is present, experienced as corporeal bits lodged inside the infant, which it can, in fantasy, expel out of itself and into the mother. If the mother has the capacity to receive such a 'bad object' into herself, to tolerate and 'contain' it, to work it over, 'metabolize' it in her mind through a capacity for 'reverie', she can return 'the object' to the infant in a thinkable form as an *alpha-element*, not a present bad object inside the infant but an idea *of* an absent object (Bion 1977).

Where Melanie Klein conceived what she called *projective identification* as an important primitive defense, Bion identified it as also the first mode of communication between mother and infant, in fact, the origin of thinking. If the mother 'gets' the infant's communication and reflects on it, it becomes a known and tolerated experience for the infant; and 'if the infant is not too persecuted or too envious, he will introject and identify with a mother who is able to think, and he will introject also his own now modified feelings' (O'Shaughnessy 1988: 179). In the less fortunate cases, an excess of bad internal objects may lead to an excess of projective identification, which may engender an endless cycle of splitting off the bad, reincorporating the attacking bad internal objects, reprojecting them, and so on. Such a person cannot use the capacity for thinking to the fullest.

It is an ingenious theory, but no more than Hume's does it tell us how judgment arises. The plausibility of both derives from a notorious ambiguity in the Humean notion of 'sense-data'. They are stimuli that are in themselves meaningless, but that are nevertheless said to be representational: they are impressions *of* an orange, or *of* the color scarlet. Like Freud's *Trieb*, they are conceived as straddling the mind–body 'frontier'. But sensations are modifications of an organism, part of the causal story of our seeing things, as are events in the brain and nervous system; sensations are not *what* I see, and they have no representational status (Rorty 1979). Thoughts are not merely caused *by* things in the world, they are *about* things in the world; intentionality cannot be captured by a causal account in terms either of what in the world is causing us to have thoughts, or of the stimuli that connect us to the world. Hume describes the experience of seeing an orange as having an orangeish mental object before the mind. He calls it a sense impression, a datum of sense, of which the idea of an orange is a pale copy. But an impression is not itself orange; rather, it is an impression *of* something that one can judge *is* orange.

Think of it this way: when we say that a chimpanzee sees an orange, we mean that something *we* identify as an orange is apparently the cause of neurological, experiential, and behavioral changes in the chimpanzee. But this causal connection does not prove that the animal has a mental experience *of* an orange, an experience that it can identify as representing an orange, a belief that it recognizes might be false. In the theory of knowledge from Hume on, the concept of a sense-datum or impression trades on an ambiguity between mere sensation, and sense-datum as a propositional 'idea' like 'the table is red', or 'there's Mama'. Sense-data in the first sense are part of the causal story of thought, but nothing more; in the second sense they cannot explain thought, since they presume it, a circularity that Wilfred Sellars (1956) referred to as 'the myth of the Given'.

Bion's theory rests on just the metaphors that need to be cashed in: sense-data are 'cast into corporeal form'; the mother transforms mental 'bits' in the infant's mind, then 'injects' them back into the infant; mind is a 'thinking apparatus', a 'container'. As in the triangulation story about mental development, communication plays a role, but Bion leaves out the essential concepts of truth and falsity, which are needed to ground the mutually interdependent concepts of my world, your world, and the world. Bion pays lip service to the idea of communication, but his theory shows us a mind isolated both from the world and from other minds in such a way that communication is not a form of dialogue or reciprocity between persons, but an invasion of body parts.

One might try to defend Bion by saying that he is drawing the picture of mind he attributes to the infant. But it is Bion who describes thoughts as corporeal bits and mechanical things, who calls thinking an apparatus, rather than a vital, ongoing, engagement between human creature and surrounding world. Like Freud and like Melanie Klein, for whom the infant naturally occupies a paranoid–schizoid position, Bion mistakenly thinks pathology is a guide to mental functioning in general. Nor can the phenomenology of thinking gone wrong yield its own explanation. Thoughts can seem to 'appear from nowhere'; they can be dissociated from each other; thinking can be stuck, repressed, constricted. But such phenomena do not warrant Bion's claim that thoughts precede thinking in the order of development. Isolated, dissociated, thoughts arise out of the activity of thinking, no matter how disordered it may be.

In saying, *contra* Bion, that thinking necessarily comes with thoughts, and that both come with the child's learning his way around the world, we are abandoning the building-block theory of judgment as hopeless. Not even symbols will provide the blocks, if by symbols we mean units of meaning prior to thinking; for, understood in the usual way, symbolizing is a sophisticated activity that again presumes judgment.

What, in the way of the mental, precedes judgment? Fantasy and primary process? Freud defined primary process as a kind of thinking in which there is 'no negation, no doubt, no degrees of certainty . . .'. Processes in the unconscious are said to obey different laws, which Freud calls 'in their totality the *primary process*' (1940: 164). In a similar vein Freud (1915a: 187) says the system *Ucs.* is characterized by '*exemption from mutual contradiction, primary process* (mobility of cathexis), *timelessness, and replacement of external by internal reality*'. And we recall Freud's saying in the passage quoted at the beginning of this chapter that, with the introduction of the reality principle, one species of thought activity was split off and kept from reality testing; Freud called this activity fantasying. In the development of mind, fantasy and its prototype, hallucination, are said to come first.

Amplifying the notion of primary process, Anna Freud (1936: 7) writes that when 'the so-called "primary process" prevails, there is no synthesis of ideas, affects are liable to displacement, opposites are not mutually exclusive and may even coincide and condensation occurs as a matter of course. The sovereign principle is . . . that of obtaining pleasure.'

The notions of primary process and fantasy run together several different questions. (1) Is there a kind of mental content—fantasy (hallucinatory wish-fulfillment)—that precedes judgment and gives rise to it? (2) Is there a sort of thinking that, while it may presume all that secondary process does, nevertheless has a peculiar kind of organization? (3) Are there some memory systems that precede the development of explicit, declarative thought, and whose contents have some of the quality Freud attributed to primary process? This last is a question for which contemporary developments in neuroscience have provided the vocabulary. (see LeDoux 1998; Westen 1999, 2002). I will be addressing only the first. I should note that some of my remarks about fantasy and primary process overlap discussions by others (e.g. Rycroft 1962; Holt 1967).

Fantasies are described by Klein and Bion as being *about* the breast, *about* having a bad breast inside, or projecting badness into another, and so on; therefore, according to my earlier argument, fantasies are intentional and representational; they presume judgment. So Bion *unintentionally* implies in saying that, where there is an excess of projective identification, omniscience may take the place of learning from experience by aid of thoughts and thinking, for he remarks that in this case 'there is therefore no psychic activity to discriminate between true and false' (1988: 181). But a creature that has no concepts of knowledge, of the true and the false, cannot think itself omniscient.

We find an idea similar to Bion's in Britton (1998: 12–13) 'A belief is a fantasy invested with the qualities of a psychic object and believing is a form of object relating . . . I think belief, as an act, is in the realm of knowledge what attachment is in the realm of love.' He adds, 'Subjective belief comes before objective validation or reality testing.' I am not sure what Britton means by 'objective validation' and 'reality testing', since presumably the infant is in some sense testing reality from the beginning—that is, learning the shape of his mother's face, how loudly he has to cry to bring her to him, or how hard he has to suck the nipple or the bottle to make the visual array before him change. So I take Britton to mean that belief, as a mental state or attitude, comes before the ideas of reality and objective validation, a view I think he shares with Bion.

Of course we can have particular beliefs we have not tested, we refuse to test, or are not aware of having. But, in general, that sense of 'belief' that relates belief to knowledge, justification, and reasoning requires, I have argued, a grasp of the concepts of the true and the false. Britton (1998: 12) himself suggests something like this when he says, 'stating that one believes something is saying that one takes it to be true but accepts the possibility that it may not be true'.

Fixity and inattentiveness are among the marks of unconscious fantasy, as is pathogenic belief. These characteristics may be rooted, furthermore, in certain developmental failures. Peter Fonagy's work (1996a, b) has recently been exploring what some of these might be. But it does not follow that belief is initially a state of certainty on the part of a creature not yet capable of doubt. Prior to their becoming conscious, fantasies are 'indifferent' to questions of truth and falsity in the sense that the fantasizer has not raised them. But this is different from the idea that fantasies can occur in a mind that lacks the ideas of truth and falsity altogether.

Is there room for primary process and fantasy in the sketch of thinking I have given ? Yes. Take primary process first. Freud himself thought of it as primary in several senses, one of which has to do with particular ways in which unconscious thoughts are organized; and this is how it has often been understood in the psychoanalytic literature. Holt (1967), for example, says that, in unconscious thinking, objects and things are classified according to attributes that would ordinarily be judged non-essential; Rapaport (1951: 708): 'Where the primary process...holds sway...everything belongs with everything that shares an attribute of it . . .'. Recent research also supports a distinction between mental organizations that group things together on the basis of different principles (Brakel et al. 2000). This research is mute on the temporal order of primary and secondary process.

Both daily life and clinical practice acquaint us with a host of ways in which the mind turns away from what it perceives and knows. To explain these and other phenomena, Freud pitted a first kind of thinking that is inherently wishful, driven by sex and aggression, against a later kind of thinking that is oriented to reality. We now have good reason for saying that the infant mind is acquainted with reality from the first, and comes to understand it *as* reality in the very process in which it becomes able to think. Primary process describes a particular organization of thoughts in a minded creature who has made all the tracks through the world to which secondary process alludes. As for fantasy, I suggest that it is an anxious spin on thinking, not its earliest stage.

6
Self-Reflections

I am taking off layer after layer, until at last . . . I reach the final,
indivisible, firm, radiant point, and this point says: I am! like a pearl
ring embedded in a shark's gory fat.

(Vladimir Nabokov, *Invitation to a Beheading*)

If then you say that in such cases the mind thinks, I would only
draw your attention to the fact that you are using a metaphor, that
here the mind is an agent in a different sense from that in which
the hand can be said to be the agent in writing.

(Ludwig Wittgenstein, *Philosophical Investigations*)

The concept of the self began its modern slide into incoherence with
Descartes. Descartes said, we recall, that I can know that I exist in any
act of first-person thinking. The act of thought itself, as expressed in
'I doubt that p' or 'I believe that p', confirms the existence of myself
as thinker. But, Descartes noted, it is the existence of myself only as
a disembodied, un-worlded mind that is so confirmed. The idea of
self, that to which the 'I' use presumably refers, must be innate.[1]

Denying innate ideas, Locke attempted to find the origin of the idea
of the self in experience. He came up empty-handed, reluctantly
claiming that in no way can we experience or intuit this mental substance. Nevertheless he invoked it to resolve what he thought was a
paradox, that a person can change while remaining the same, and to
explain the coherence of mental states that personal identity presumes.
Though unobservable, there is a substance, Locke claimed, that unites
one's mental states.

---

[1] See Wittgenstein (1958) for a discussion of the idea that 'I' does not refer at all.

Hume picked up Locke's question: What can we observe that accounts for personal identity?, and answered, more rigorously, Nothing. With Descartes in mind, Hume (1951: 252) wrote:

There are some philosophers, who imagine we are every moment intimately conscious of what we call our Self; that we feel its existence and its continuance in existence; and are certain, beyond the evidence of a demonstration, both of its perfect identity and simplicity . . . For my part, when I enter most intimately into what I call *myself*, I always stumble on some particular perception or other . . . I never can catch myself.

When I introspect, Hume is pointing out, I can catch various representations of myself: myself having breakfast this morning, myself as a professor, myself as a 3-year-old child. But I cannot catch the 'I' who is doing the representing. Hume concluded that the self is an illusion; that what we call the self is nothing but 'a bundle of perceptions'.

Hume himself knew that this is unsatisfactory, at the very least because the perceptions in this bundle are mine, not yours. This points to the puzzling fact that self-knowledge cannot, in the ordinary case, come by means of identifying criteria. How do I know that *I* am the person now speaking or thinking this thought?[2] Surely not in the way that I know that the person across the street is Tom; for, no matter how exhaustive the criteria, I can go on asking: 'But how do I know that I am the person so described?'[3]

We began with the first-person point of view, and that seems to be the very thing of which we can give no account. Descartes and Locke held that the self is a mental substance; Hume, that, so far as he could tell, there may be no self at all. But all three philosophers took first-person thinking itself for granted.[4] If, instead of asking straight away, 'What is the self', we ask what is required for someone to be able to think a first-person thought in the first place, to make what I earlier

---

[2] Ricoeur (1992) distinguishes two senses of 'identity': *idem*, which contrasts with change, and *ipse*, which contrasts with otherness. My identity as a self implies that I am distinct from other persons; it does not imply some unchanging core of personality.

[3] The literature on this subject is enormous. See in particular Cassam (1994); see also Nagel (1983).

[4] Kant (1949) argued that all experience is necessarily experience *for* a subject. Whatever thoughts I have I must be capable of recognizing as my thoughts. Acknowledging Hume, Kant says that in 'the synthetic unity of apperception', I am conscious of myself not as I appear to myself, but merely *that* I am.

referred to as judgments, we are led to a different view; for we see that one must have already learned to distinguish oneself from others. He knows that one person can occupy different places at different times while remaining the same person; that you are you whether you are here or there, whether it is now or then, and so with me; that nobody else traces exactly my trajectory in space and time. First-person thinking can be engaged in only by a creature who recognizes some of his beliefs and desires as elements in his continuing history. My knowing that I exist, and that the thought is mine, not yours, comes through the same engagements with the world and other creatures in it that yield judgements. I have learned, we might say, the grammatical rule that 'I' refers to the one who uses it. But grasping that rule is a complex process.

I conclude that, if by 'self' we mean a subject, a thinker who can perform Descartes's initial act of self-reflection, an agent who can doubt, reflect, and argue, then one becomes a self through those very understandings that allow him to speak for himself. First-person thinking requires a long and intricate pre-history—in the world and with other persons. We generate puzzles about what the 'I' refers to, or how I know I am 'I', or the same 'I' from one thought and one moment to the next, when we forget that there are background conditions for thought.

Knowing that I am the subject of this thought does not require a kind of perceptual act in which I spot myself as the thinking subject. Nor does knowing that it is p I believe typically require an inward glance. In the simplest case I believe that p,—for example, that it is raining—because I see or hear that it is. And, if I am asked whether I believe that it is raining, I look at the world again. In this respect, beliefs are, as Gareth Evans (1982) puts it, 'transparent to the world'. Of course, if p is complicated, I may need to examine a whole network of attitudes in which p is enmeshed; in this sense I look inward. But the network itself faces the world.

Our concept of the first person is contingent on the world, and on particular ways the world is.[5] Were we creatures of a very different kind, creatures who, as the philosophers' puzzles imagine, continually fuse or fission, the constraints that are built into our concept would also

---

[5] Campbell (1994) explores these conditions at length.

be different. Harry Frankfurt's idea, to which I turn shortly, that beliefs and desires can occur as a succession of separate moments, may fit creatures other than ourselves; but it does not fit a creature who is constantly constructing a narrative in which he figures in the first person. First-person thinking is necessarily accompanied by a sense of oneself as a historical continuant, one who, when he is explicitly conscious of believing that p, knows that belief as his. We understand ourselves as thinking, desiring subjects only to the extent that we grasp our behavior and our thoughts as parts of a unified activity. Where this breaks down to a drastic extent, as it does in various forms of psycho-pathology, or as a result of trauma, so does one's sense of self.

While other animals may be conscious, reflexive self-consciousness, the capacity not merely to have a thought but to know that I do, is peculiar to the human animal, and a condition for many of the things we value most about ourselves. Reflexive self-consciousness allows us not merely to change in appropriate response to the world around us, or to be changed—rabbits too can run for the shade—but to take a peculiarly active hand in that change. It allows us to reflect on what we do, construct ideals against which we measure our own behavior, take responsibility for our actions, and become more integrated creatures. A Cartesian idea of the self takes its unity for granted. On a historical, developmental view, the unity of the self is not a given but an ideal, a matter of more closely integrating relatively disparate elements.

So Harry Frankfurt (1988) holds. But the concept of the self in his work still has an unfortunately Cartesian cast. Frankfurt links integration of the self with autonomy, which I think is right. But, viewing integration as strictly an internal matter of how parts of the self are arranged with respect to each other, he neglects those aspects of the 'I' with which I began: the subject's historical nature and his relations with the objective world of which he is a part. I believe this is why Frankfurt's idea of autonomy is finally unsatisfactory.

A person has autonomy, Frankfurt argues, if he is ruled by desires that are really his. A desire is mine if it is a desire I choose to have. At first sight this is paradoxical, Frankfurt admits, for how can one choose one's own desires? Who is doing the choosing, and by what is he moved?

To answer this, Frankfurt invoked in earlier essays simply a distinction between first- and second-order desires. First-order desires are the ones I find in myself. They have as their objects the doing or the having of something. But we also form second-order desires—that is, desires that takes one's own desires as their target, as when I want not to want to smoke, or not to feel envy, or to be moved by gratitude. The agent wants to have a desire that he does not have, or he wants an existing desire to be effective in moving him to action. Frankfurt calls a second-order desire of the latter sort a 'second-order volition', a case of wanting a first-order desire to be one's *will*. Since a first-order desire is something we merely find in ourselves, it is only our second-order desires, Frankfurt argued, those endorsed by us, that begin to define us as autonomous agents.

Frankfurt came to think, however, that the mere fact that one desire occupies a higher level is insufficient to give it greater authority: the ordering does not allow us to determine 'where (if anywhere) the person himself stands'. To fill this need Frankfurt added the idea of a desire that is not merely second order but also wholehearted, 'resounding' throughout the other orders of desire. The hierarchical picture now is this. At the bottom are our 'elementary motivational tendencies'. These are not truly ours; they become so only if, at a second level of desire, we choose to make them so. Through our volitional attitudes we structure the contour of our will, determining what we will love and care about wholeheartedly at yet a third level.

The wholehearted carer is the one who acts freely because he wholeheartedly *identifies* with his own volitions, and because the volitions with which he identifies depend, in a certain sense, on nothing outside himself. Frankfurt asks us to consider an erroneous carer, the person who, in his example, 'cares' about not stepping on cracks in the sidewalk. Undoubtedly Paul, as we will call him, is committing an error. But how should we describe it? The intuitive answer, Frankfurt says, is that Paul cares about something that is not worth caring about.

What makes something worth caring about? Frankfurt wants to answer this without appealing to anything outside the person himself. His strategy is to say that what makes something worth one's caring about it is either the fact that it is antecedently important to the agent, or that caring about it is itself what is important to him. Paul's caring is presumably the second sort of error. It lies in the fact that 'it is not important to [him] to make avoiding the cracks in the sidewalk important to himself' (Frankfurt 1988: 93).

But how does Frankfurt know, to begin with, that Paul has made any kind of error? Presumably because we know enough about our fellow creatures to recognize that behaviors like Paul's cannot summon into play the interests, talents, skills, and pleasures that make something worth caring about. In this respect, avoiding cracks is different, for example, from gardening, playing the violin, climbing the Geiger, activities that one can learn to do better and that yield beauty and excitement as the reward. These are pursuits, furthermore, in which others engage: one can compete, fail, but also excel, winning as one does the admiration of others who also appreciate gardens, music, or mountains. Avoiding cracks in the sidewalk, we suspect, is motivated not by some love or caring through which the self flourishes, but from an anxiety that constricts and cripples it.

Here I have implicitly invoked a different answer from Frankfurt's to the question of what makes something worth caring about. I have said that it is a function, in part, of properties of the activity and of ourselves and agents, and is often something for which we can give reasons, reasons that are intelligible to others. (It may, of course, turn out that the reasons we give are not really the ones that move us.) For example, if I believe that Paul intentionally avoids the cracks in the sidewalk, then I have to assume there are reasons why he cares as he does. So I might ask him to tell me more, in the way I sometimes ask someone who likes a painting that leaves me cold what he sees in it. We cannot argue others into liking Braque or Brahms, but there are many things we can do to try to get them to hear or see what we do, for example, pointing out aspects of the object, setting it in comparison with others, explaining some of the principles of its composition. —All this I count as 'giving reasons'. —Or, I might suppose that avoiding cracks belongs to a culture that is alien to me, and try, like the anthropologist, to discover the network of practices, beliefs, desires, values, and so on, that illumine it as a ritual with a communal sense. If either of these two strategies is successful, then I have no reason for thinking Paul has made an error.

Suppose he cannot tell me why he does what he does; he may even say he does not know; he just has to do it. Then I might try, like the psychoanalyst rather than the anthropologist, to understand what it is Paul fears. If he is moved by irrational fears, fears that make no sense even to him, then his problem is not, as Frankfurt says, that he is vainly

straining against some limit of caring in himself, but that some unconscious motive interferes with his knowing what it is he 'cares' about, or
indeed from caring about it in a way that forwards his own projects.

Paul's behavior seems not to be an instance of caring at all in the
sense Frankfurt invites us to consider. He wants to distinguish caring as
one kind of orientation toward the future, not to be confused with liking
something or wanting it: the person who cares '*identifies* with what he
cares about in the sense that he makes himself vulnerable to losses and
susceptible to benefits . . . regarding it' (1988: 83). 'Caring' then has
the sense of to care for, to take care of, as in 'take under one's wing'. The
wishes both to avoid something dangerous, and to engage in something one finds gratifying and pleasurable, help explain what we do, in
some sense, voluntarily. But to the extent that the motivation involves
unconscious fears or conflicts, the more we begin to question just how
voluntary the action is. Typically, in cases like Paul's, the motivation is
not caring in Frankfurt's sense, but fear that something terrible will
happen if one disobeys the prohibition one has constructed.

Frankfurt's account of the erroneous carer, I am saying, misses the
mark. And so does his account of the wholeheartedness in which
autonomy is said to consist. Frankfurt suggests that Martin Luther
proclaiming 'Here I stand! I can do no other' is an instance of freedom;
that, paradoxically, the 'free' action embodies this peculiar kind of
necessity. To be sure, Frankfurt makes clear, it is not the necessity of the
alcoholic who wants to stop drinking but is constrained by a desire he
disowns. Yet his words at least tell us that Luther also is acting under
constraint, if 'only because he does not really want to do it'. This
'volitional necessity' is then both self-imposed, yet imposed involun-
tarily, since 'otherwise it will be impossible to account for the fact that
[he] cannot extricate himself from it merely at will . . . A person's will
may be no less truly his own when it is not by his own voluntary doing
that he cares as he does' (1988: 87–9). In saying 'I can do no other', Luther
is expressing the conclusion of a complex process of caring in which
a first-order desire that he has simply found in himself is then endorsed
by him, finally becoming a wholehearted desire with which he identifies and to which, in this sense, he binds himself.

We are captive to what we love at both the first and the third levels,
but there is a crucial difference between them, Frankfurt continues, in
that our first-order desires are given, contingent, dependent on the

world, while our wholehearted volitions, coming about as they do through our second-level identifications with our own desires, are authentically ours. Frankfurt thus argues against Kant that love, and not only reason, can make us free; for, when a person acts in ways demanded by his wholehearted love, his volitions depend entirely on the inherent nature of his will. Freedom can then consist precisely in this peculiar kind of necessity. Hence the importance of what we care about; for, if someone is somehow mistaken about his own cares, or if he cares or tries to care about things that do not allow him to care wholeheartedly, he will not be able to constitute himself as an autonomous agent.

But I do not think that Frankfurt has resolved the paradoxes. As he presents him, the self who constitutes himself *as* a self is as elusive and mysterious as Descartes's thinker; for the second level of the hierarchy seems to introduce a sort of uncontingent, transcendent ego, a *causa sui*, a self conceived as standing in relation to the various mental attitudes that constitute his mind as a conductor to an orchestra. We glimpse this ego in the contrast Frankfurt draws between human caring and the way in which, according to one theological doctrine, God cares. God's love is 'entirely arbitrary and unmotivated—absolutely sovereign, and in no way conditioned by the worthiness of its objects'. While it may be possible for an omnipotent being 'to love altogether freely and without conditions or restrictions of any kind', such a love is not possible for us (Frankfurt 1988: 94). Yet, when we care about something not because we think it is important independently of our caring about it, Frankfurt continues, but just because the caring is itself important to us, then in this respect we come as close as we can to the love of God.

Consider again Frankfurt's ideas about caring. Surely, if God's carings are dependent on nothing outside Himself, it is because in His case alone we can make no sense of the distinction between the desired and the objectively desirable. Nor can we make sense, I think, of a caring that is absolutely unmotivated. Desires that one can avow *are* tuned to something that *is* beyond the agent. Luther 'can do no other' because, on reflection, and given everything he believes, knows, and values, this action is what he most wants to do. He acts in accord with desire but also reason, in the form of reflection and thought; for reason is among the mental activities that have shaped his desire. A reasoning agent considers not only the harmony among his own desires, but also the validity of the beliefs to which they are linked, and the nature of the things or situations in the world, when such there are, that are the targets of his desires. He asks himself 'Do I really want it?', 'What is it that I want?', and 'Is it worth having?' Frankfurt apparently takes for granted the contentious claim that about values there can be no fact of the matter, nor such a thing as justification.

Our beliefs are oriented in the first place toward the world. That is also the reach of desire. Bishop Butler's classic refutation of Hobbes consisted in pointing out that 'the very idea of interested pursuit presupposes particular passions and appetites, since the very idea of interest or happiness consists in this that an appetite or affection enjoys its object. Take away these affections and you leave self-love absolutely nothing at all to employ itself about' (Butler 1950: 14). If, parallel to the question 'Do I believe that p' I am asked 'Do I want p?' or 'Do I value p', I may look to my own attitudes, seeing, for example, whether this desire is consistent with something else I want. But at some point I check the object of desire itself.

John wants, or thinks he wants, to become president of the First National Bank. Reflecting on whether he really wants it will require him to investigate the bank, and what being president would involve. Appraising one's own desires will also, ideally, involve making explicit hidden, unconscious beliefs that are constraining one's desires. Jim is reluctant to buy the house he loves. On investigation he realizes that this is because he basically does not believe that he should have something so wonderful. Now that he is aware of having it, he can ask himself whether this belief is one he really honors.

How would Luther justify his stand? Frankfurt has given us, we recall, two alternatives: a person can claim that 'the thing is independently important to him' or that 'caring about it is itself something which is important to him' (Frankfurt 1988: 93). But these alternatives omit the most obvious way in which we justify the things we care about, the way that Frankfurt explicitly bypasses: we appeal to the worth of what we care about. Luther might have publicly justified his decision by arguing the importance of his action to the life of the Church, or by repeating his reasons for thinking that the practice of Indulgences was corrupting. Luther's primary interest is not himself but the world, of course, the world as he sees it. And he is likely to become clearer about his choice if he investigates the world as well as himself.

What is importantly right in Frankfurt's emerging picture is its emphasis on the contingency of the self. Who we are is a complicated interaction between the contingent and the uncontingent, the given and the chosen, the not-I, or the not-yet-I, and the I. But the emphasis on contingency is not radical enough. The self as a kind of hierarchy seems right. But everything in the hierarchy is dependent on something else. So it is not clear in Frankfurt's account how our contingent desires are related to the self-governing self that may—given whole-hearted caring—emerge. It is not clear who the *he* is who determines what his will is to be, nor how he determines it.

The errors in Frankfurt's account of autonomy come right at the start in his claim that every first-order belief and desire of a person is atomic. Frankfurt (1988: 83) writes:

> Desires and beliefs can occur in a life which consists merely of a succession of separate moments, none of which the agent recognizes as elements in his continuing history . . . The moments in the life of a person who cares about something, however, are not merely linked inherently by formal relations of sequentiality. The person necessarily binds them together.

From the first-person point of view, mental content seems to be atomic: I can know that I am thinking 'I am hungry', 'I hope I am making myself clear', 'I wonder what the weather will be like in New York tomorrow', without consciously being aware of anything beyond this moment. But, if we approach the mind from a third-person point of view, we see that understanding another's mind begins with our experience of him in a material world we share; and what I learn from that experience informs me of some general features of my own mind. It is from this third-person point of view that we can see from this third-person point of view that mental contents are not atomic, but take their meaning, in part from their neighbors, in a sort of holistic web. If you mean what I think you do when you say 'It's raining outside', you must believe something like 'Rain is wet', 'It's not a sunny day at the moment', and so on. And the same is true of me. Furthermore, there are normative, or rational, constraints on meaning. For example, if you believe that it is raining right now on Avenue B, and you mean what I do by those words, then you cannot also believe that it is not raining right now on Avenue B.

If it were true that desires and beliefs were linked merely 'by formal relations of sequentiality', then integration would be possible only given some further capacity or faculty, perhaps the one Frankfurt calls volition. But, on the contrary, the content of any thought is constituted in part by its relations with other thoughts, memories, and perceptions, and much of the integration, or of the defensive holding apart, requires no person to do the binding. When one mental attitude or state changes, so then will the others to which it is most closely related.

To account for desires that are truly mine requires a structure that is essentially temporal: it changes over time such that desires, thoughts, memories, many of them unconscious, are continually rewoven into the fabric of the mind. The structure also yields an ongoing narrative: persons are creatures who have stories to tell, and ideally these stories are open to change.

Something else that Frankfurt omits is crucial to selfhood: our relations to other persons. In Shakespeare, Montaigne, and Pascal, the authentic self is what one is in and for oneself, as distinct from what one affects for others (Trilling 1972). These writers do not question that often it is expedient, even moral, to present a false face to the world. But they worry that doing so may lead to self-betrayal oneself, to become the mask one has affected. Such worries are among the reasons we should be as suspicious of second-order desires as of any others.

Distinguishing the true from the false self is partly a matter of different kinds of identifications, not with our own desires but with other persons; and of different ways in which these identifications are and are not integrated into the mental fabric as a whole. For example: out of unconscious guilt, one may identify with a mother one sees as impotent and fragile, perhaps in the belief that one is oneself responsible for her injuries, or the fear of causing her further harm. Such an identification obstructs knowing, and pursuing, what one wants. Or, as a defense against terror, one identifies with the aggressor in a way that fractures one's own moral values. In such cases we construct a false self.

Mark Epstein (1995: 73) writes: 'The crumbling of the false self occurs through awareness of its manifestations, not through the substitution of some underlying "truer" personality.' And Winnicott (1965: 148): 'There is but little point in formulating a True Self idea except for the purpose of trying to understand the False Self, because it does no more than collect together the details of aliveness.'

Winnicott connects the idea of a True Self with the spontaneous gesture. The child makes a gesture—a novel use of words, a facial expression, an interesting bodily doing or action—that is prompted not by the need to be what the mother wants the child to be in that moment, but by the child's own desire. The good-enough mother meets the child's gesture with one of her own that is attuned to the child's feeling. There is a moment of dialogue rather than obedient pretense or parroting. The mother who is not good enough substitutes her own gesture with which the infant is to comply. One's sense of oneself as an alive creature in the world, coherent through time, who invests things with meaning and can initiate activity, comes, early in life, through being recognized as such a creature by another.

We are familiar in religious writings with the idea that we become more ourselves the less self there is in us. Frankfurt (1988: 89) asks: 'How are we to understand the paradox that a person may be enhanced and liberated through being seized, made captive, and overcome? Why is it we find ourselves to be most fully realized... when—through reason or love—we have lost or escaped from ourselves?' I have been saying that we cannot answer that without bringing in the external world, which is where desire finds its first-order objects. We discover what they are only through action and interaction with them, in the process discovering—making—ourselves. Love that is relatively unambivalent explores its worldly objects with interest. It tends to establish coherent patterns of behavior, informed at once by knowledge, desire, and valuing, patterns that we identify as ourselves: 'I am a pianist—an Israeli—a mother.'

Unfortunately we are not all equally such lovers. Freud calls the openness to the world the reality principle. It is necessary to the formation of 'the ego'—the 'I'. Freud also knew that this openness is often painful; we have various strategies, conscious and not so conscious, more and less successful but never wholly so, for sealing ourselves off from the world and for closing the world out. Our emotional and our perceptual systems orient us towards other persons and reality; so we cannot totally deny either reason or love. Yet we try. These movements have a rending effect, for the wheeling inwards that produces fantasy forms psychological constellations that are relatively separate from the psychological fabric as a whole.

The line between what is my self and what is not, between the authentic and the false self, cannot be drawn with the external world on the other side.

PART III
Problems of the Self

7
Irrationality and Self-Transcendence

What interested me was not a philosophy of the free man ... but a technique: I hoped to discover the hinge where our will meets and moves with destiny, and where discipline strengthens, instead of restraining, our nature.

(Marguerite Yourcenar, *Memoirs of Hadrian*)

A Model for Irrationality

Various sorts of irrationality pose no conceptual problem. If I make a decision or form a belief on the basis of what you consider to be insufficient evidence, you may think I am irrational; but I am not, or not necessarily, if I genuinely think the evidence is sufficient. But suppose that I make a decision or hold onto a belief on the basis of what I myself consider to be insufficient evidence; or am paralyzed by an anxiety for which I myself cannot find a good reason, or deceive myself about my own beliefs and feelings; or that I have committed myself, or think I have, to a course of action on which, though neither a change of mind nor anything outside myself interferes, I do not follow through. It does not matter whether the contrary beliefs or the desires that are behind my conflicted state are conscious or unconscious. Either way there is an internal incoherence that threatens my very being as a minded agent.

The paradox arises from the fact that if, as we have said, the content of a mental state is constrained by its normative relations with other mental states in a holistic mental network, then rationality is not an optional feature of the mind but among the very conditions of its existence. How can we render this normative constraint consistent with the evident existence of irrationality? By making use of a particular aspect of the distinction between reasons and causes. In the typically rational case, Davidson argues, the reasons why an agent performs an action are also among the causes of his doing it: James looks out the window *because* he wants to see if it is raining. In the irrational case, however, James does something because he wants to, but he himself does not consider his wanting to be a reason, that is, a *good* reason, for doing it: his wanting the chocolate sundae causes him to have it; but he had resolved to lose weight, and, as a means toward that end, not to eat the chocolate sundaes that he craves.

Davidson (1982: 300) asks us to consider first a case in which the cause and the effect occur in different minds: 'wishing to have you enter my garden, I grow a beautiful flower there. You crave a look at my flower and enter my garden. My desire caused your craving and action, but my desire was not a reason for your craving, nor a reason on which you acted. (Perhaps you did not even know about my wish.)'

This is a straightforward instance of intentional behavior on the part of two persons, an instance whose interest lies in the fact that *A* provides *B* with a reason for acting in such a way that *A*'s end is achieved, even though *B* does not do what she does with *A*'s end in mind. *B* acts for a reason, but it is not *A*'s reason, which moves *B* merely as a cause.

Though there is, of course, neither paradox nor necessarily any irrationality in the two-person case, nevertheless it makes clear, Davidson (1982: 305) continues, that 'mental phenomena may cause other mental phenomena without being reasons for them . . . and still keep their character as mental, provided cause and effect are adequately seg-regated'; and so the two-person case suggests a strategy for dealing with irrationality in the solitary mind. Making sense of someone requires us to attribute to her various maxims of rationality, including the one Davidson calls 'the principle of continence', or doing that which, all things considered, one thinks it best to do. The irrational agent is not one who altogether lacks this principle—such an *agent* there cannot be—but one who manages to bracket it off to one side. In the rational case, two explanatory schemes, reason—in the form of interlocking beliefs and desires, conscious and unconscious—and cause, coincide; in the irrational case, a gap opens between the two schemes. When such non-rational mental causation is at work, the single mind may to some extent resemble a duality of minds, or a mind that is, as we familiarly say, divided within itself.

As an example of such a 'bracketing', Davidson gives a variant on an incident in Freud's case history (1909) of the Rat Man. A man walking in a park stumbles on a branch. Thinking it may be dangerous to others, he removes the stick and throws it in a hedge beside the path. On his way home, however, it occurs to him that the branch may be dangerously projecting from the hedge, so he returns to the park and replaces the branch in the road. Both actions are rational in and of themselves, for in each the man acts in the light of a reason, a belief–desire complex that is necessary to explain the action. If he had not had these reasons, he would not have done what he did; so the reason in each case is also a cause.

The irrationality consists not in doing either of these actions, nor even in doing both, but in the fact that in returning to the park to replace the stick the man intentionally ignores not only his own initial reasons for removing it, but also the principle of continence. He has a motive for ignoring it—namely, that he wants—perhaps for very strong unconscious reasons—to restore the branch to its original position. Presumably he believes he will be less anxious or somehow happier if he does. But this motive enters his reasoning twice over, first in overruling his own reasons for removing the stick, and second in overruling the principle of continence. In brief: the irrational agent wishes not to act on his judgment of what it would be best to do, all things considered, and this wish causes him to put the principle of continence to the side.

Such an explanation of irrationality draws a boundary, then, between two groups of largely overlapping mental states, only one of which contains the principle of continence. Desire, the sort of thing that can be a reason, causes one to do something for which there can be no *good reason*—namely, to act without considering the consequences of one's action, or without taking all the consequences one has considered into account. There can be no good reason for putting the principle of continence to one side, since it is a principle constitutive of reason itself. The postulated boundary, Davidson remarks, is not to be thought of necessarily as a line between conscious and unconscious mental states but merely as a conceptual aid in giving a coherent description of certain genuine irrationalities.

Freud also recognizes the need for something like the principle of continence in describing irrationality. It is because he does that he is moved in *The Ego and the Id* to revise his topography of the mind (Freud 1923). Earlier he had envisioned internal or intra-psychic conflict as taking place between consciousness and the system unconscious, one 'self' knowing but not wanting to know, the other genuinely ignorant, with 'the censor' located more or less on the side of consciousness. But he came to see that among the facts not pictured by this model is that 'he repressed' does not merely happen to be unconscious, but is actively kept out of consciousness, and by a repressing agency that is itself unconscious of what it does. So, partly for this reason, Freud introduces the structures 'id', 'ego', and 'super-ego', to cut across the conscious/unconscious divide. Much of the ego ('das Ich') is repressed; but the ego is also that which acknowledges and attempts to reconcile conflicting beliefs and desires, and in doing so sometimes represses. Freud's 'ego' is that agent who—because he or she implicitly acknowledges such principles of rationality as we have posited—can be said to repress and to 'split'.

In the following passage from a late essay 'Splitting of the Ego in the Process of Defence', Freud (1940: 275–6) writes:

He [the child] replies to the conflict with two contrary reactions, both of which are valid and effective. On the one hand, with the help of certain mechanisms he rejects reality . . . on the other hand, in the same breath he recognizes the danger of reality, takes over the fear of that danger as a pathological symptom and tries subsequently to divest himself of the fear . . . But everything has to be paid for in one way or another, and this success is achieved at the price of a rift in the ego which never heals but which increases as time goes on . . .

So far, then, Davidson and Freud agree in saying, first, that interpretation requires us to think of the mind as largely rational; second, that the irrational agent is able to hold beliefs or desires that he knows to be incompatible and incoherent apart; and, third, that irrationality of this sort forces us to think of that aspect of ourselves we call the mind as divided. Like Davidson, Freud, at least some of the time, endorses an idea of the divided mind according to which desire, appetite, and belief are strands in a mental fabric of a generally rational character. Freud and Davidson agree in a view of irrationality quite different from Plato's division of the soul into a rational rider and two horses of a different color.

Let us see how Freud (1909: 189–90) tells the story of the man and the stick that we looked at earlier:

One day, when he was out with her [his lady] in a boat and there was a stiff breeze blowing, he was obliged to make her put on his cap, because a command had been formulated in his mind that *nothing must happen to her*. This was a kind of *obsession for protecting*, and it bore other fruit besides this . . . On the day of her departure he knocked his foot against a stone lying in the road, and was *obliged* to put it out of the way by the side of the road, because the idea struck him that her carriage would be driving along the same road in a few hours' time and might come to grief against this stone. But a few minutes later it occurred to him that this was absurd, and he was *obliged* to go back and replace the stone in its original position on the road.

The man's narrative begins with a tale of dreadful punishment involving rats, a tale by which he is obsessed and which he vividly imagines happening to his father and his 'lady'. At first this obsession presents itself as 'just a thought'; but the fact that his feelings about this 'thought' are fascination and anxious guilt suggests that he is envisioning this punishment for his father and his lady, and that for him it is as if what he envisions were about to come true. Freud links this incident to the rat obsession, to others of the man's obsessively violent thoughts, and to his bizarre compulsion to work until late at night, followed by his masturbating in front of the mirror. This last compulsion Freud analyzes, in part, as the acting-out of a fantasy that the father he knows is dead is alive, and properly horrified by the man's defiantly exhibitionistic behavior.

Recall that on Davidson's analysis the irrationality of the man's behavior with the stick/stone enters at the point at which he ignores his own best all-things-considered judgment. I would say, instead, that in this instance there is no such judgment at all. Davidson's account may more or less fit something that happened at some time in the agent's past. But, whereas Davidson construes the division merely as a logical necessity of our analysis, I construe it as a full-fledged psychological event, perhaps recurring repeatedly with the recurrence of the traumatic situation, and creating a kind of psychological fault that persists over time, consolidating habits and processes that have rendered the agent incapable of genuine all-things-considered judgments in certain situations now. (By a 'genuine' all-things-considered judgment I mean one that sees, is able appropriately to weigh, and attempts to take account of the relevant facts. It is not, of course, an uttering of the formula 'this is my all-things-considered judgment'.) On the fuller concept of division that I am urging, the split-off structure precedes the irrational act; it is not another description of it in philosophical language, but an empirical explanation of how it can occur.

In the typical cases of 'Freudian' irrationality the split-off mental structures are created around relatively early anxiety. I imagine that the anxiety situation that initiates a split-off structure is chronic—for example, a threatening ever-present father and a seductive mother—and that the response to the anxiety situation is one on which the child comes habitually to rely. Then habits of misperception begins to settle; the exiled structure begins to crystallize and consolidate.

It is such a structure that Freud's interpretation reveals behind the Rat Man's act of putting the stone back in the road. The structure contains his early hatred toward his father, perceptions of him as very powerful, a 'projection' of his own anger onto his father, perhaps misperceived as angry toward him, self-deceptive feelings of his own innocence, certain early beliefs (for example, that his thoughts are visible to others and endowed with a kind of magical power), and the tendency to see other persons either as objects of his desire or impediments to it, a tendency that has presumably governed his relations with the world from early childhood. The structure as a whole is marked by confusions between past and present, between what is the case and what one wishes were the case, even between what are genuinely pleasurable thoughts and what are thoughts that are 'pleasurable' only in that they help ward off anxiety.

Thus early on the 'split' takes on character, dividing fragmentary impressions, together with fantasies formed as a defense against them, on the one hand, from, on the other, more occurrent perceptions in potential conflict with the fantasy structure. What started out as a wishful belief acquires the force and structure of a habit, a way of acting, a way also of perceiving, that reinforces the initial avoidance. Old fears, old memories, both veridical and false, that might have a very different meaning now if one reflected on them, are preserved. And, given that the imagination works in the associative way it does, more and more situations may come to remind the fantasizer of what he does not want to confront. It is such a process Freud describes when he sometimes speak of 'the unconscious' as pulling conscious thoughts into its vortex.

Freud saw a crucial link between early childhood anxiety and repression. Such there may be, simply because in childhood one is so vulnerable, and not yet able to deal with dangers in the world by taking the appropriate actions. A kind of psychic flight, or looking away, together with what Freud sometimes calls hallucinatory wish-fulfillment, may be the only defense at the child's disposal. Furthermore, he is not yet able to put many of his anxieties into words, or not in a way that renders them sensitive to conscious judgment.

Davidson's account of irrationality is meant to be highly abstract; he explicitly says that he is not giving the psychological detail that would be required in a given case. But, as applied to the episode of the stone in the road, and others like it, Davidson's account does not do justice to the fact that the divisions of the self are neither of the same temporal order, nor the same order of agency: in the main structure, occurrent beliefs and desires open to evidence, and subject to revision in the ordinary way, along with the capacity for all-things-considered judgments; in the substructure, beliefs and desires that are embalmed, increasingly alien to those of the present, and inappropriate in the light of present experience. When this substructure is activated, judgment is temporarily clouded, or in abeyance. Freud's story reminds us that beliefs and desires are formed against an affective background and enmeshed in defensive habits, often of long standing.

Rationality and Self-Transcendence

There are, of course, trivial cases of non-rational mental causation, as when the thought of forks reminds me of spoons, a caveat that already opens the door to processes of various sorts that escape the paradigm of practical reason. But far more interesting, Davidson (1982: 305) remarks,

is a form of self-criticism and reform that we tend to hold in high esteem, and that has often been thought to be the very essence of rationality and the source of freedom . . . What I have in mind is a special kind of second-order desire or value, and the actions it can touch off. This happens when a person forms a positive or negative judgment of some of his own desires, and he acts to change these desires. From the point of view of the changed desire, there is no reason for the change—the reason comes from an independent source, and is based on further, and partly contrary, considerations.

This is what I call the problem of self-transcendence. The mere having of incompatible desires is not the situation we are considering. In such a dilemma the agent looks more closely at what each desire entails and decides, if possible, which is the more important. Conflict of this sort can be difficult, even paralyzing, but it is not conceptually puzzling. Nor is it if, moved by a desire of which I know you disapprove, I find I value your approval more than the satisfaction of my desire and so, only to please you, act when you are around as you would like me to. At the extreme, I am then like the woman in Purcell's song who wants to fly from love's sickness but finds that she is herself her own fever.

Where the incontinent person remains fevered, however, betraying her own values or desires, and so, herself, the reasonable person instead gathers her conflicting desires under a banner to which she can give her allegiance, and acts accordingly. Yet how does she manage it? How can one who desires to have different wants find a point of leverage on her wanting self? If the incontinent act is irrational, it also seems to be, once one is in the state from which the act issues, inevitable.

Let us say that I want to stop smoking. It is hard, for after all I am, I say to myself, a smoker. Of course this is not quite right: I smoke, and if I say to myself that I am a smoker, this is true only as a description of what I do in fact. So Sartre reminds us when he tells us that the kind of 'being' that thinking creatures have is not fixed, obdurate, like the 'being' of a stone, but rather a horizon of possibilities from which I continually choose. Since smoking does not befall me, as fits of coughing may, but is an activity I intentionally, if habitually, perform, we are in the domain sketched above in which someone wants to change her own effective wants. Clearly there is little available in the mental network closest to the desire to smoke that allows me to put my countervailing desire straightaway into effect. This is my problem. And berating myself every time I fail in my resolve is only apt to intensify the unease that prompts me to smoke in the first place.

Yet there are things I can do, and do intentionally. For example, if I have been wanting to go white-water canoeing, an enterprise that I incidentally know will reduce the chance of smoking, and even perhaps the desire, to a minimum, I might sign on for such a trip, hoping to use it as an occasion to change my ways. I play the gardener to myself by appealing to a desire x, the enacting of which will set a causal chain in motion that may result in the satisfaction of a desire y that I am not able to achieve directly. Or, if I am tired of my tendency to procrastinate writing letters, I might thrust myself into a position that permits no delay. Or, if I would like to stop getting into wrangles over trivial matters, I might try diverting my own attention or the conversation when I see a wrangle in the offing.

Though just which strategy will be effective will vary from case to case and person to person, the strategies agree in that one does something intentionally in the hope of changing a pattern of behavior of which the targeted desire is a part. If I am successful, I will have done something I wanted to do; and my wanting was not irrelevant to my success. But to say *tout court* that I stopped smoking because I wanted to would not do justice to the complexity of the causal story, which includes intermediate and devious goals, and things that more or less happened to me along the way.

Changing bad habits like the ones in these examples is hard enough. But it is child's play compared with the difficulty of changing a characterological trait like the tendency to envy another's good, or to spoil his pleasure in his beautiful flower because it is not one's own, or to take one's own misfortunes more seriously than one thinks seemly, and so on. Here we are up against things that most truly reveal who we are and before which we feel all the more helpless.

Let us revert to the gardener who seeks to lead his neighbor voluntarily into his garden by giving her a goal that will coincidentally achieve his own. His hope is that, once she is in his garden and has come to know him, the gardener, sometimes her reasons will be his reasons in that he and she will enter into ventures that require the sharing of many goals. Towards this end he may have taken the trouble to learn that it is gardens and not, for example, antique cars to which she is susceptible, daffodils and not roses. So, like the gardener, the envious person may need to become a good detective, noting in what circumstance the envious wish takes hold, what anxieties emerge if he does not act on it, what old conflicts the circumstance reminds him of, and so on.

We might summarize the difference between the irrationally incontinent and the rationally continent persons in this way: Emma, who falls into incontinence, and Isabel, who manages to avoid it, are at the same fork in the woods. Emma takes a familiar path marked out by habits of various kinds, towards an end that will incidentally (or not so incidentally) yield a familiar self-dismay; but Isabel finds incentives to lead her in a different direction, one that may begin to put new habits into play. Only if we construe habit as more mindless than it is, and intention as less a matter of habit and of practice, should Isabel's behavior puzzle us. Dewey remarks that we tend to think of bad habits and dispositions as forces outside ourselves. We tell ourselves, truly, that the habit was not deliberately formed. 'And how can anything be deeply ourselves which developed accidentally, without set intention?' But all habits are 'demands for certain kinds of activity; and they constitute the self. In any intelligible sense of the word will, they *are* will. They form our effective desires and they furnish us with our working capacities' (Dewey 1944: 24–5).

The paradigm of practical reasoning takes desire itself as a given. Often, however, desire grows slowly from what one does. By definition desire is a state of want, yet for what may not be clear. Habits are the material of desire; desire rises to the surface on a sea of practice. The so-called first order desires are just those fully formed desires that, unopposed by older desires more deeply ingrained in our behavior, come with the means for acting on them attached. Dewey (1944: 30) goes on to say: 'If we could form a correct idea without a new habit, then possibly we could carry it out irrespective of habit. But a wish gets a definite form only in connection with an idea, and an idea gets consistency and shape only when it has a habit in back of it.'

A half-formed idea may go no further; or it may. What is expressed in a work of art, for example, is not fully present in the mind before the work is created, but comes to be in the act of expression itself. Dewey (1934: 71) writes: 'What is expressed will be neither the past events that have exercized their shaping influence nor yet the literal existing occasion. It will be . . . an intimate union of the features of present existence with the values that past experience has incorporated into the personality.'

Dewey means this description to apply to any meaningful activity, for it 'is the fate of a living creature . . . that it cannot secure what belongs to it without an adventure in a world that as a whole it does not

8

Freedom and Understanding

It is quite true what Philosophy says: that Life must be understood backwards. But that makes one forget the other saying: that it must be lived forwards.

(Sören Kierkegaard, *Works of Love*)

One mark of a successful analysis, it has been said, is that one comes to see the inevitability of what she has done. In a sense that seems right. Someone who relentlessly regrets not having become a singer, or feels guilty for not having been kinder to her aging mother, has probably not yet gone far enough in the analytic work. It is not the regret itself that makes us suspect this but its relentless character.

The remark is puzzling, however; for, if what we did was inevitable, then surely what we will do is equally so; and, in this case, why should we ever consider, reflect, deliberate on, choose, which course to take? Yet we do sometimes do these things, and it would be impossible to convince most of us that we should just let nature have its way with us, or stay in bed all day like Oblomov, the character in Goncharev's novel. In doing so he is not beyond choice, but making a choice, however peculiar. Still, it is sometimes suggested, all choice is illusory.

Freud (1916: 28) writes: 'are (there) occurrences, however small, which drop out of the universal concatenation of events . . . If anyone makes a breach of this kind of determinism of natural events at a single point, it means he has overthrown the whole *Weltanschauung of science*.'

The 'concatenation' in question is presumably causal. Determinism, here, is the thesis that all events, including all mental events, are caused by prior events in the natural order of things. Freud (1919: 236) assumes that from this thesis about causality it follows that there is no such thing as freedom: 'there are also all the unfulfilled but possible futures to which we still like to cling in phantasy, all the strivings which adverse external circumstances have crushed, and all our suppressed acts of volition which nourish in us the illusion of Free Will.' What is the illusion? That we can affect the future by what we do? But obviously we can. It is anxiety about this that drives many people to think of themselves as playthings in the hands of destiny. We are as prone to exaggerating our helplessness as our power.

Freud was not alone in thinking causality and freedom incompatible. Spinoza held that men believe themselves to be free only because they are unconscious of the causes whereby their actions are determined. Like all others, mental phenomena belong to the natural order, and are caused. In this sense, determinism holds sway. But a number of philosophers, among them Locke, Hobbes, Hume, Kant, Mill, even Spinoza himself, and many others in our own time, have argued, each in different ways, that causal determinism is both compatible with freedom, and a necessary condition for it. Spinoza claims, as Freud does implicitly as well, that we become more free as we become more aware of the causes of our actions. When this happens the causes no longer move us from outside ourselves but from within: we become self-ruled, autonomous. I will follow philosophical tradition in calling such arguments compatibilist, and the arguments for freedom, libertarian.

My arguments will overlap with some of theirs. I hope to show that there are no good arguments of a general nature to establish that freedom is an empty concept. Freud and psychoanalysis describe many limitations on freedom, not by showing that everything we do and think is caused, not by showing us the reach of unconscious mentality, but by showing us psychological factors that make inroads on the ability to choose, suggesting at the same time ways in which the domain of freedom for any one person might be enlarged.

Mind, Reason, Cause

We often describe what we and others do in a mentalistic or inten-tionalist language that contains the concepts of wish, belief, desire, fear, emotion, feeling, motive, reason, intention, and so on, both conscious *and* unconscious. In the paradigm case, desires interlock with beliefs to form a reason. I want to see the new ballet by Thomasson; I believe that the San Francisco Ballet is performing it on Saturday night; so

I decide to go to San Francisco on Saturday night. Beliefs and desires interlock in ways that are logical, or rational, in an important sense of the word. For example, it is reasonable for you to attempt to avoid someone if you believe he is dangerous. It is reasonable even though the belief may not be true. It is reasonable for you to take an umbrella, given that you believe it may rain; and so on. This is of course a highly schematic account of reasons, which in any instance are going to be much more complicated.

In the absence of internal conflict and competing reasons, a particular reason in the narrow sense of a belief–desire complex becomes your intention. And, in the absence of unexpected obstacles, your intention causes an action. An action, typically performed in the real, external world, is something done for a reason in this sense. It is not merely a piece of behavior, like lurching into your neighbor when the subway stops, but behavior that is engaged intentionally. Agents are creatures who perform actions, not all, but some of the time. Creatures who are agents in this sense we call *moral* agents in the belief that someone who does things for reasons can sometimes be held responsible for her actions, responsible not merely in the sense that she caused the event in question to happen but that she did so volitionally, of her own free will, knowing to some extent what she was doing, and in possession of moral standards of some sort.

Reason is an essentially normative notion: if you believe it is reasonable for you, to do given what you want, what you believe about getting it, what else you want, and what you know about the world and yourself, then you believe that x is what you ought, as a rational person, to do. Only the behavior of persons calls for explanations that are normative in this way.

An intention is not just any wish or desire that you have *but the one on which you will act if nothing gets in your way*. You act as you do *because* you have this intention. In an ideally rational case, the intention has been considered; competing desires and troubling consequences have been weighed, and you believe the action you intend is possible for you to accomplish; for if you believe it is impossible to fly, you cannot *intend* to fly, though you may wish you could. Wish and choice differ in that the latter, ideally at least, takes into account one's own competing wishes, together with some relatively realistic assessment of both the means of achieving what one wants and some of the likely consequences.

Often we see that something we might otherwise want is discordant with other desires that are stronger.

Because it requires cognitive and emotional sophistication, *choice* enters our explanatory vocabulary later than do *wish* and *want*. A baby wants to have the rattle; she does not choose to have it, even though she may look at two rattles and go for one rather than the other. A 2-year-old may express the wish to become a physicist, like his father, but he cannot choose to do so because he cannot know what achieving these ends would mean. A young child may wish to wish to kill her brother, even choose to give him a push, but she is not capable of *choosing to kill* him until she has the concept of death. Choice demands a conceptual repertoire that wish does not.

The range of volitional doings that are open to a creature depends on what she is capable of envisioning and understanding, the descriptions that are available to her under which she sees the world. Oedipus is guilty of murder because he intended to kill the man at the crossroads. But he did not know that the man he killed was his father, so he is not guilty *patricide*. (We intend to do what we do only under certain descriptions. Oedipus did not recognize his victim *as* his father, so patricide was not part of his intention.) The breadth of descriptions available to any of us at any time determines how richly meaningful the world can be, and what intentions it is possible for us to have. The frequent claim that language separates us from world flies in the face of the fact that, on the contrary, language and cognitive development vastly expand the range of possible perceptions, the myriad ways in which we can see what we see, and expands also, therefore, the range of our choices and intentions.

We can begin to see how many are the ways in which the capacity to choose can be compromised: by a rigidity of perception that restricts what one sees, casting it into a too-familiar mold; by undue anxiety about the act of choosing itself; by constrictions on wanting and on one's ability to know what one wants; by an unwillingness, or a characterological inability, to appraise one's desires and to weigh them against each other; and so on.

What is the relation between choice and cause? A partial answer is that choices are caused by reasons in the form of mental processes and states. Among the causes of Janet's giving this concert is her choice to do so, which is itself the result of earlier choices she has made, for example, to practice, to go to Julliard, not to become a doctor. Those choices were also the effects of perceptions, beliefs, and desires, which reach back further. For some of these beliefs and desires there are in turn reasons, both conscious and unconscious: the wish to become a concert pianist may have its causal roots in Janet's earlier desire to please her father, together with her fear that, were she become a doctor, like him, she would jeopardize their relationship. At some point, however, reason-explanations run out.

In sum: choices are not uncaused events, but events *among whose* causes are reasons. Of course a great many causes of any choice are not reasons,—in Janet's case: her Aunt Jane's encouragement, her father's promises and threats, her tyrannical teacher, all of which are external to Janet. The effects of these external 'objects' and events on Janet depend on how she interprets them. Nevertheless they are themselves external. Other people can do things that cause one pain and that one reads, perhaps incorrectly, as punishment; but other people can also be truly perceived as punishing. They seduce, betray, and abandon. Psychic reality is not where the inner object world begins. This is the point of Winnicott's distinction between need and wish, the maternal holding environment, and the baby's wishes that arise within it.

The skeptic about freedom may say: *I'll grant that among the causes of Janet's giving this concert are mental events like choice itself, belief, desire, and so on. But choices are enmeshed in a material world that helps determine the choices we make and that we have not itself chosen.*

This is so. But how does it deny choice? Enmeshment tells us, on the contrary, that, to exercise choice fully in any instance, a moral agent must be able to appraise the world as he finds it, relatively free of illusion, delusion, self-deception, reactions that are triggered by old, outdated alarms, and constricting, self-imposed, rules. No one is ever a perfect agent; but there are degrees.

The skeptic pursues: *A free choice is one that was itself chosen. But, as you have yourself indicated, choice initiates in something we were simply given. So then there can be no free choice.*

The idea of a free choice can seem to require that one be moved by nothing of which one is not entirely the author; yet to divorce action from motivation, if one could, would empty of meaning not only the concept of choice, but also the concepts of action, agent, and agency. Without my past, my character, my upbringing, my culture, my habits, beliefs, and desires, all of which are causal factors that have helped construct my motives, who would *I* be? (The idea of an *acte gratuit*, an arbitrary act, which defined freedom for Gide, in fact obliterates the agent.) So Hume (1951) argues in distinguishing what he called liberty of indifference from *liberty of spontaneity*. Liberty of indifference would obtain were there uncaused events, which is not the case. But this empty sense of liberty, Hume goes on to say, is not the one we need to anchor moral agency. That presumes, rather, liberty of spontaneity, or the ability to do what we want to do. This liberty we sometimes have. And it does not require that every strand in the choosing process was itself chosen.

Think, for example, about belief, and the role of belief in choice. In the absence of belief there can be no choice. But do we choose our beliefs? Normally, and ideally, no. In fact, the more rational we are, the more our beliefs are determined not by what we want but by what we find. I believe the ballet will be performed on Friday night because I read about it in the newspaper. I believe you are a danger to me because you have threatened me. (If I believe it because I am inclined to see danger everywhere, my belief is to that extent not rational.) David Wiggins (1987: 271) writes: 'the libertarian ought to be content to allow the world to dictate to the free man . . . how the world is.' And Susan Wolf (1990: 119–20): 'Since human agents live within a world of facts already established, knowledge *of* the world, and therefore knowledge necessarily shaped by the world, in which they must act is, for the most part, promotive of freedom and responsibility rather than inimical to it.'

The skeptic: *Free choice, choice, it doesn't matter. I believe that instead of choice we will one day be talking only about genes, neuro-transmitters, hormones, and so on. Those will be our basic explanatory concepts of human behavior. This is the sense in which choice is an illusion.*

If the skeptic could establish that there are no mental events (processes, experiences), it would follow that there are no choices, since choice is a meaningful concept only for creatures with minds. Molecules combine, volcanoes erupt, mosquitos transmit malaria, but not by their choice. And, though neuro-transmitters are involved in choice, it would be a category mistake to speak of neuro-transmitters as agents of choice. The concept of choice is essentially tied to the concept of mind, such that, were 'reason' found to be superfluous as an explanatory concept, so would choice; the concept would in that sense be illusory.

The skeptic about free will is not apt to claim explicitly that there are no mental events. He argues instead that everything we now say in the language of mind we will one day be able to put into the language strictly of body. This is, I believe, the hidden assumption in Freud's argument against free will. He speaks as if the problem were causality; but causality is a problem only if mental sorts of things, like reasons, cannot be causes; that is, only if our behavior can be entirely explained in the same way as the movements of that part of nature that is unthinking. This is why I began with the reason/cause distinction.

Only a century ago we would have heard the claim that there are minds, and that minds are not merely bodies, as a metaphysical claim about the numbers and kinds of substances in the world. Few philosophers nowadays are dualists of that sort. We believe that all mental events have bodily, neurophysiological substrates; minds are not entities of a special kind. Nevertheless some bodily entities are 'minded' in the sense that adequately to describe and explain their doings requires a mentalistic as well as a physicalist language. Our understanding of human behavior requires two mutually irreducible languages, a language of body, or matter, and a language of mind.

The world for which the language of mind is indispensable is the world in which people marry, tell lies, play chess, feel guilt, perform a *ronde de jambe*, try to avoid prophecies, wish they had not done what they did, and so on. All these descriptions are shorthand for a large number of more specific activities to which the concepts of thought, belief, desire, are indispensable. For example: If someone can accurately be described as performing a *ronde de jambe*, she must know something about ballet, have the concept of that particular movement, and want to be doing just that movement. The language of mind is needed not only for explaining a lot of human behavior, but also for describing it: Maria is moving her leg that way because she wants to perform a *ronde de jambe* and believes that is how to do it. What is Maria doing? Performing a *ronde de jambe*.

Hence the argument of those philosophers who, following Wittgenstein, have insisted that reason explanations are not causal explanations. Unlike the first, causal explanations are not teleological: they do not appeal to aims, goals, intentions. Furthermore, cause and effect are distinct phenomena—the earth quakes and the picture on the wall falls down; the mosquito bites and the child gets malaria— whereas reasons simply, it can be argued, describe or redescribe an action.

Reasons do describe, but not *simply*: Oedipus killed an old man at the crossroads, Oedipus murdered an old man at the crossroads, Oedipus committed patricide at the crossroads. Reasons, in the form of beliefs, desires, memories, fantasies, and so on, are not identical with the actions they explain: the *ronde de jambe*, the murder. It is true, and important, that reason explanations have a peculiar pattern: they set an event in the context of a particular human life, character, way of looking at the world, culture, practice, or set of practices. And reason explanations must take into account the subjectivity of the agent, the fact that her behavior can be adequately described only through appealing to her own first-person point of view. This is why there is no clear line to mark off Maria's performing the *ronde de jambe* from the social–psychological context that helps constitute her gesture as a *ronde de jambe*; and why the explanations for two actions that may look alike can never be the same. We may describe them both as a *ronde de jambe* or a patricide, but these are labels, unhelpful to us as interpreters of particular persons.

And this is why there can be laws of only the roughest sorts that generalize from particular motives, explanations, actions. Reason explanations, unlike causal explanations that do not 'rationalize', are at the same time justificatory, in that finding the reasons for someone's action means finding what was to be said for it *from her point of view*. On all these differences turn the familiar distinctions between *Verklärung* and *Verstehen*, between the natural and hermeneutic 'sciences'.

So why, in the face of such differences, insist that reasons are causes? Because one might have all the reasons for lifting one's leg, murdering an old man, yet not do it, or do it, but not for those reasons. It is to capture this aspect of the relationship between reason and action that we call reasons a species of cause. I did what I did *because* I had those reasons (Davidson 1980*a*).

But can we say that reasons are causes if we assume, with Hume, that every particular causal relation implies the existence of a general 'law' that covers it? How could we accommodate this assumption to the view of reason explanations put forth above according to which, in important ways, no two reason explanations can be the same? In the following way. Grant that every mentalistic description picks out an entity, or process, or event that can in theory be picked out also by a physicalist vocabulary. In this sense we would be granting that all mental events and phenomena are physical phenomena, but again, not *merely*. It is not that an action is a composite of mental and physical components, but rather that the language for describing what happened as, on the one hand, an action, and, on the other hand, a mere bit of behavior, is fundamentally and irreducibly different. Perhaps there are even physical laws linking up types of events, physically described. But from phenomena described in a mentalistic language, we can generalize only roughly. (Davidson 1980b).

Here are the three things that might be meant by the reducibility of the mental to the physical: (1) every mental event or state is a material event or state, though the converse is not the case (not every material event or state is mental); (2) there are laws correlating all the explanations stated in a psychological language with explanations in a physical language, laws that themselves belong to the physical sciences; (3) science can and should get along without the language of mind altogether.

We can grant, I am saying, that the first claim is true, without granting the second, which is highly unlikely. Take my earlier example of my going to the new ballet by Thomasson, which I decided to do at noon on Thursday. Call this decision a thought about *pi*. The identity theorist will presumably claim that this mental event is identical with some noontime brain process p (having definite physical features x, y, and z). But it is not remotely plausible that every thought about *pi* is a brain process with these physical features. Even so simple a mental phenomenon as my thought about going to this particular ballet on this particular day reaches into a unique complex of memories, associations, and so on. For another, 'there is no reason to suppose intelligent creatures elsewhere in the universe would need to share our neurophysiology or even our biochemistry in order to think about *pi*. It is not even plausible that every *human thought about pi*, or even every *thought of Mary's about pi*, is identical with a brain process falling into a class specifiable solely in terms of the physical features of its members (Dennett 1978: 253). For these reasons most philosophers now think that token–token identity is the best sort of mind–body identity theory we can have.

I am arguing for a kind of explanatory dualism on the mind–body question that might resemble what Mark Solms calls 'dual-aspect monism', about which he says:

Dual-aspect monism accepts that we are made of only one type of stuff . . . but it also suggests that this stuff is *perceived* in two different ways. The important point to grasp about this otherwise straightforward position is that it implies that *in our essence* we are *neither* mental nor physical beings . . . that brain is made of stuff that *appears* 'physical' when viewed from the outside (as an object) and 'mental' when viewed from the inside (as a subject). (Solms and Turnbull 2002: 56)

The mind–body dualism, Solms concludes, is an artifact of perception.

But this claim rests on a miscast distinction between 'inside' and 'outside'. My perception of you as attempting to seduce me is from the 'outside', but I atttribute to you, perhaps truly, a first-person perspective that allows me to describe you as having seductive thoughts and intentions. Intentions and decisions are not merely 'inner' phenomena; nor do we wear them on our sleeves. But, if nothing gets in the way and if they really are our intentions, then they are expressed in the external world. We believe that the person who insists, even as he helps himself to the third cream-puff, that above all he wants to lose weight is self-deceived, or deeply confused.

An explanatory dualism about mind and body does not necessarily imply that mind and body are merely linguistic entities. Rather: there is a real world in which we live and with which we are in touch, some of whose characteristics require us to use the language of mind; for others the language of body alone will do. In the development of the universe as a whole, body almost certainly came first, as it does also in the development of every individual human being. But this does not mean that body, or the language of body, is metaphysically privileged. It does not mean that really, *objectively*, we are only bodies in motion, and minds only from our *subjective* point of view. Where would we have to be standing, so to speak, to make that claim? As speakers, thinkers, investigators, we are subjects; can we say, as subjects, that we are really only objects? No; for in making claims we are necessarily acting as subjects. The claim that there are minds is then as much a conceptual claim as it is empirical in that no discoveries could persuade us to abandon 'mind' as fundamental to our understanding of human life.

   In the area of mind–body connections, research is teaching us about the effects of things like hormonal deficiency, genes, and neuro-transmitters, on mood and thought, of constitutional disposition on emotion, of emotion on cognition, about the effects of unconscious registrations on what we think and do. In describing the effect of emotion on behavior, the relations between conscious and unconscious mental events, the distinction between the articulable and the mute, we see a slide where before we saw a chasm. Undoubtedly we are on the threshold of many more discoveries about what we sometimes call mind–body interactions. Furthermore, we may think someone is an agent with regard to a particular deed, and later find out we were wrong. But, from the fact that we often make mistakes about agency, it does not follow that there is no such thing and that we are always in error.

   Isaiah Berlin says that advances in psycho-physiology might some day convince us that determinism is true, and libertarianism false. He presents this, that is, as an empirical issue. But he grants that, if this were to happen, a change in our conceptual scheme would be required that would exceed any that have gone before. Praise and blame would no longer be based on the presumption that the agent could have acted differently, but would have the function only of changing his future behavior; predicates like brave, generous, virtuous, which now imply something about the kinds of choices the person has made, would be transformed into descriptions on the order of 'pretty', 'muscular', 'agile'; our current talk of choosing, intending, deciding, would have to be replaced by a repertoire of concepts it is impossible now to imagine (Berlin 1998). This in itself is no argument against determinism, Berlin remarks, but a consequence of which its proponents may not be aware.

   Yet, in elaborating how extensive these conceptual changes would be, Berlin is in fact arguing against determinism; for, if adjectives like 'brave', 'generous', and 'virtuous' were to go, so would 'honest', 'reason-able', 'truthful'. *No* mental predicates would survive. So we are back to reducibility. And if no empirical discoveries could persuade us to abandon the concept of mind, then, because of the conceptual links between freedom and mind, freedom, too, is indispensable. The domain of reasons is also, and necessarily, the domain of choice, decision, agency. Reason and reasons, mind, belief and desire, choice, freedom, moral agency and moral responsibility, are all of a piece; banish one and out go the others. Where we presume of another creature that she has a mind something like our own, we also presume that she is, to some extent, a free agent; though both presumptions are, to an extent, defeasible. The 'revision in our conceptual scheme' to which Berlin alludes would not be the sort that makes understanding between creatures from different cultures particularly difficult. It would not require a change from one conceptual scheme to another, but, impossibly, evacuating ourselves from the domain of reason altogether.

Some years ago Peter Strawson (1974) argued for a version of libertarianism along similar lines. About ourselves and each other we know that we sometimes have intentions and do what we do deliberately. We also know that we often make mistakes, have accidents, do things that have harmful consequences that we did not intend, take aim at the right person but hit the wrong one because we were not careful enough, aim at the wrong person mistaking him for the right person. save the person's life who later murders our friend, and so on. When someone has harmed us and we assume it was intentional, we are naturally angry and resentful; but, if we discover it was unintentional in some way, we exonerate, or perhaps forgive.

But sometimes we may judge a person to be so mentally deficient or otherwise incapacitated that we think it inappropriate to hold him responsible at all; he is not subject to moral judgment; he is not an agent, we implicitly say. Could this always be our attitude towards other persons? Strawson asks. Can we seriously imagine adopting such an attitude as a result of a conviction that determinism is true? Is it possible that we might some day find evidence sufficient to persuade us that a non-reactive attitude would be, in all cases, the rational stance?

We cannot answer this, Strawson argues, without considering what we mean by rationality. Rationality is a feature of human beings, who are by nature bound together by ties of need, love, obligation, commitment, responsibility. Never to have a reactive attitude towards others would mean not treating another fully as a person, able to engage with oneself in the special ways that people do with each other. It would entail an intolerable isolation. To try to regard *oneself* with such non-reactive objectivity, I might add, would be self-annihilating. 'When we do in fact adopt [a non-reactive] attitude in a particular case,' Strawson (1974: 83) concludes, 'our doing so is not the consequence of a theoretical conviction which might be expressed as "Determinism is the case", but is a consequence of our abandoning, for different reasons in different cases, the ordinary inter-personal attitudes'. This is a different way of putting my earlier argument: the language of mind, which is presumed by the moral concepts, and a strictly physicalist language are mutually irreducible; both are required for the living of our human lives and for the understanding of human action.

In sum: there are no facts of a general, metaphysical nature to rule freedom out. Psychoanalysis shows us not that free will is an illusion, but that our peculiarly human capacity for choice is constrained by phenomena that are equally peculiar to us as symbol-using creatures. Psychological defenses sometimes operate as givens that are, in the moment, beyond our will, governing how we choose and who we are.

D. Shapiro (2000: 30) writes:

> The basic model of defense as a control structure that denies access to consciousness is not an adequate conception of the self-regulative, or defense, process. As soon as one recognizes the dynamics of character as a self-regulating system, the nature of defense appears in a new light. The defense mechanisms can then be seen simply as features of the system. These processes are not 'used' by the person, as is sometimes said; they are processes, constituents of the person.

A defense 'mechanism' is something I can find in myself. But in coming to understand what it attempts to ward off, I may disable the mechanism.

There is no such thing as *absolute* freedom; or, rather, we cannot coherently articulate such a concept. There are degrees of freedom, and no clear line to be drawn between innocence and guilt. Spinoza (1963: 75) writes: 'There is in no mind absolute or free will, but the mind is determined for willing this or that by a cause which is determined in its turn by another cause . . . In the same manner it may be shown that there cannot be found in the mind an absolute faculty of understanding, desiring, loving, etc.' Only a Substance, defined by Spinoza as something that contains all its own determinants within itself, is *absolutely* free; and the only such things are mind *in general*, body *in general*, and God, not particular minds, bodies, or agents.

Freedom and Forgiveness

Speaking for the underground man, Dostoevski (1972: 20) writes: 'I should probably have been unable to do anything with my generosity; neither forgive, because the person who offended me might have been following the laws of nature, and you can't forgive the laws of nature; nor forget, because even if it was according to the laws of nature, it was still an affront.' The underground man's dilemma arises from the fact that he looks at the world, as he must, from his own first-person point of view, feeling resentment and forgiveness and demanding appropriate objects for his feelings, yet he denies there are any such.

Earlier I invoked Strawson's distinction between a reactive attitude that regards the miscreant as a full member of the human community, a person whom we, often appropriately, resent, blame, hold responsible, and forgive; and a non-reactive attitude in which such attitudes are inappropriate. Strawson calls the latter 'objective'. But we might call an attitude towards a creature, oneself or another, 'objective', in a different sense of the word, to the degree that it acknowledges her as a person with a first-person point of view. Doing this effectively is to be able to identify with her. The attitude is both objective and reactive, and in taking it we may be able to forgive her. Empathy is called for even if the person is oneself, for example, if the deed to be forgiven took place some time ago, when one was in an important sense *a different person*. Just as it takes an imaginative stretch to put oneself in the position of another, so may it also if the person is oneself.

The following newspaper story nicely illustrates reactive objectivity. The defendant in a murder trial had intended to rob a convenience store run by a friend of his named Beers. Gross had approached the store with a gun held at his side, out of sight. Beers buzzed him in. Gross raised his gun and started shooting. The first shot hit Beers in the abdomen. Gross continued to fire. Three shots missed, but a fourth struck Beers in his chest. Pleading, 'Oh God, please, no,' Beers stumbled into the back office. Gross followed, and, to get a better angle, shifted the gun from his right hand to his left. Beers begged for mercy. Gross shot him in the face and fled from the store.

Since the entire crime had been recorded by an unseen camera in the corner of the store, Gross's deeds were not in question. Furthermore he confessed. A few weeks later, after viewing the tape of the murder, the prosecutor told a reporter for the local newspaper: 'There isn't a jury in this world . . . that would not recommend the ultimate penalty in this case, the death penalty.'

At the beginning of the trial the defense attorney, Hill, conceded to the jury that he had no case; but he went on to say, 'we have substantial evidence to preserve his life'. He said that his task as a defense attorney was 'to make sense out of the nonsensical. . . . I wanted to get the jury to walk in Jeremy's shoes.' Hill had hired a 'mitigation specialist' who helped the attorneys find witnesses, and worked to gain their trust. The specialist spent a year and a half interviewing people who had in some way touched Gross's life, including his mother. What emerged during the penalty phase of the trial was a finely detailed story of child-hood disaster.

The jurors quickly found Gross guilty of first-degree murder. But the penalty phase of the trial lasted for five more days, after which the jurors voted for a life sentence without parole rather than death, even though all twelve had said before the trial that they were not in prin-ciple opposed to the death penalty. Later, one of the jurors explained her change of heart by saying that she had been struck with the thought that Gross could have been her son, and that she could not understand parents who treated their child as he had been treated. Another reported that what she had earlier interpreted as Gross's indifference she now saw instead as his feelings of shame. Another said, 'I began to think not that there's an excuse for what happened, but I had an understanding of his torment.' Hill and the mitigation expert had managed to give the jurors a sense of the context of Gross's deed so that he was no longer merely an instance of a moral principle violated, but an individual person, with whom they could identify.

Susan Nieman (2002: 3) suggests that we think of evil as 'absolute wrongdoing that leaves no room for account or justification'. That is of course right if 'to account for' just means 'to justify'. But, taking in its other sense, 'to explain', or, in the case of human agency, 'to render intelligible', raises a question. For presumably only moral agents can do evil; and to recognize someone as moral agent is to assume that he is in some basic way similar to us, and so, in principle, intelligible. Perhaps the point is that we can make no more sense of the idea of *absolute* wrongdoing than we can of *absolute* free will.

If to understand is to forgive, then I suggest that the understanding in question is this reactive objectivity. Of course you may neither want nor be able to forgive me; I may have to do that for myself. Forgiveability depends on the one to be forgiven; forgiving on the giver. Earlier I said that a part of wisdom consists in seeing the inevitability of the past. I asked: but if the past was inevitable, why is not the future also?

My answer has been that there is some degree of choice in both cases. One's past actions were not, in truth, inevitable, if that means there was no choice. 'What is inevitable doesn't depend on whether or not determinism reigns, but on whether or not there are steps we can take . . . to avoid the foreseen harm' (Dennett 2003: 156).

We are not always mistaken in thinking we are responsible agents. Nor are we ever free of intrapsychic conflict. But we may be relatively so in certain areas of our lives, and more so in others than we have been. We make mistakes in both directions: we often believe, falsely, that we are the sole agents of our misfortune; we often fail to see the agency we have. We cannot change the past, but we can come to understand it differently, which may change how we live our lives now, precisely because we are the sort of 'objects' in the universe that have minds, reflect, and make choices.

9
Valuing Emotions

I fear that the animals regard man as a creature of their own kind which has in a highly dangerous fashion lost its healthy animal reason—as the mad animal, as the laughing animal, as the weeping animal, as the unhappy animal.

(Friedrich Nietzsche, *The Gay Science*)

Most who have written on the emotions, the manner of human life, seem to have dealt not with natural things which follow the general laws of nature, but with things which are outside the sphere of nature: they seem to have conceived man in nature as a kingdom within a kingdom. For they believe that man disturbs rather than follows the course of nature, and that he has absolute power in his actions, and is not determined in them by anything but himself.

(Benedictus de Spinoza, *The Ethics*)

Until recently the emotions were consigned to a small backyard of the mental visited chiefly by philosophers. Aristotle named the features of the emotions, set the questions, that continue to guide inquiry: the relations among emotion, belief, and desire, between emotion and action; the place in emotion of bodily arousal and physiological expression; the connection of emotion with pain and pleasure. Aristotle was the first to ask: Can emotions be said to be rational or irrational? Do they have intentional objects? Are we passive or active in regard to them? Are they in or out of our control? Are they educable?

Then somewhere in the 1960s the subject heated up. Philosophers again were in the vanguard, but they were now joined by psychologists, neuroscientists, and, of course, psychoanalysts, who, having long lamented their lack of a coherent theory of the emotions, suddenly acquired many allies in the task of constructing one. In philosophy the movement began with challenges to the traditional distinction between reason and passion, attempting to rescue the emotions from the irrational and a-rational by construing them as some combination of belief, judgment, appraisal, or evaluation, together with desire. But philosophers now writing on the emotions generally agree that, while cognition often plays an essential, constitutive role in the emotions, it does not always; and in any case cannot, even with the addition of desire, give us a general theory.

It may be that none is possible. Paul Griffiths (1997) suggests that the concept of emotion may resemble the concept of sublunary objects in Aristotle's day: there are such objects, but they have nothing especially in common to distinguish them from other arbitrary collections.[1] We do not yet know how to sort emotions, feelings, moods; mental states like puzzlement, curiosity, hope, pessimism, concern; conditions we describe by saying something like 'I feel stupid', or 'I feel that something isn't quite right between you two'; desire, pleasure, and pain. Love alone calls up a variety of related but different affections, among them: lust, friendship, marital love, maternal love, compassion, *eros*, and *agape*. And each of these terms no more than gestures at a whole affective world.

My aim in this chapter is to show that emotions are quintessentially subjective states that nevertheless have important objective and public aspects. They are subjective in that the content of an emotion can be given only in the telling of a particular individual's life story; they identify, as I say at the end of the chapter, what she cares about. They are objective first of all as appraisals of reality. In human beings an emotional state typically contains a sophisticated cognitive component in the form of belief. When this is so, then, like belief, an emotion can be rationally assessed. Second, emotions are orientations to the world that show up how things matter to us, revealing the world in its relation to us, and ourselves in relation to the world. This is not to say that our emotions are always properly tuned. I discuss this obvious fact in

---

[1] On Griffiths's view the category of emotion subsumes three different kinds of psychological state: socially sustained pretenses, 'irruptive motivational complexes' that require higher cognition, and affect program responses such as fear and anger. Some of these emotion categories, like anger, themselves reflect these fractures. By socially sustained pretenses Griffiths (1997: 245) means a kind of 'disclaimed action,' like 'falling in love,' which is the adoption of a social role that permits the performance of certain behaviors.

'Self-Knowledge and Self-Discovery'. But they are educable. Finally, we communicate our emotions to others, and expand our emotional repertoire through these communications.

At a later point in this chapter I briefly discuss the difference between emotion and feeling. For now I will mark the distinction in terms of consciousness: emotional processes may be going on of which we are not consciously aware; feelings, however, though we may not know just what the feeling is, are always conscious, that is to say, *felt*.

Belief and Emotion

Like beliefs and desires, the emotions figure in our ordinary everyday explanations of human experience and behavior. Stripped down, our explanations often go something like this: Maria slapped you because she is angry with you, and she is angry *because* you insulted her, or so she thinks. Hans hid from his father because he was frightened of him, and he was frightened *because* his father was going to punish him, or so Hans thought.

Abbreviated though they are, these little stories make clear that emotions typically have causal relations with what we desire, what we believe, and what we do. Though we do not always act on our emotions: we stay our hand, or the impulse to slap or to hide does not arise in the first place. So overt behavior cannot be made a necessary condition for the presence of emotion. And the full content of an emotion-laden experience is typically far more complex than these little stories suggest.

For example: Maria's anger on this occasion may be related to her urgent wish to be esteemed, her exquisite sensitivity to insult, a sensitivity that sets a horizon against which she perceives, and misperceives, herself and others. But she may once have had good reason to feel that somehow she is deficient, say if throughout her childhood her father consistently treated her with contempt. That earlier relationship makes her vulnerability to insult intelligible, even though her responses may be out of touch with the present. This might be just the beginning of a potentially endless narrative, the telling of which, furthermore, will inform Maria herself of the emotion's content.

Our emotions are causally linked both to other 'inner' states like beliefs and desires, and also to the world around us: Maria may have correctly perceived that her father treated her with contempt. At least in human beings with relatively developed conceptual capacities, an emotion is part of a complex causal nexus that relates emotions to other emotions, to other mental states such as beliefs and desires, dispositions to organize our experience in certain ways, perceptions, and to the external world, the whole of which forms a certain disposition to act. The causal connections go every which way: from beliefs and desires to emotions, from emotions to emotions, from emotions to world, from world to emotion, from mind to body, and from body to mind. Note that the emotion forms a *disposition* to act; whether one does act depends on other factors.

Emotions differ with respect to their degree of cognitive sophistication; but where an emotion is constituted partly from beliefs, they help identify the emotion as this particular emotion. If Toni is proud, it must be the case that she *believes* she has done well; if Sarah feels guilty, she believes that, by her own lights, she has done something wrong. The content of the emotion may be unconscious: Sarah may not know what she feels guilty about, or she may fasten on something relatively innocent that obscures the guilt's real object. But in sophisticated emotions like pride and guilt, beliefs are necessarily present.

Freud (1909: 175–6) acknowledges the conceptual connection between belief and emotion in writing about the Rat Man's guilt: 'When there is a *mésalliance*... between an affect and its ideational content... a layman will say that the affect is too great for the occasion—that it is exaggerated.... On the contrary, the [analytic] physician says: "No. The affect is justified." The sense of guilt [for example] is not in itself open to further criticism but it belongs to some other content, which is unknown *(unconscious) and which requires to be looked for.*' I take Freud to be saying not that the Rat Man has done something for which he quite properly feels guilt, but for which he believes he has; and it is this cluster of beliefs that makes the feeling of guilt intelligible, to the Rat Man, if he can articulate them, and to others.

Where beliefs and perceptions are partially constitutive of it, the emotion is subject, like belief itself, to error, education, and rational appraisal. Beliefs can be true or false, reasonable or unreasonable, wishful or realistic; they can be tested, appraised, and adjusted in the light of reason. So also the emotions that draw upon them. The Rat Man may come to see that he has confused a murderous wish with an act of murder, or that of course he felt angry, given what he now, retrospectively, can see about his father. Or, say I am aware of becoming angry with Jason because he did not call me when he promised to. A day later, still silence. Unexamined, anger may take over. But suppose I ask myself what it is I believe about Jason that is making me angry. That he has forgotten me? Not likely. I remind myself of my susceptibility to feeling forgotten. I also recall that making phone calls on this trip will be difficult for Jason. The emotion fades.[2]

Perhaps because emotions are processes that begin out of conscious awareness, it often seems as if they simply *happen* to us. But this is true only to an extent and in some circumstances. In both psychoanalytic therapy and certain meditative practices, one learns to become aware of an emotion ever earlier in the process of arousal, to appraise the emotion before acting on it, and to question the way the world looks *in the light of* what one feels.[3] Both practices are about altering those basic attitudes which, like an undue sensitivity to humiliation, dispose one to certain painful and constricting emotions.

I have been talking about those emotions that have a strong cognitive component. But the emotions run a gamut from primitive rat fear to the intricacy of Marcel's jealousy or Emma Bovary's boredom. Because of our greater cognitive capacity, our emotional repertoire is far greater than a lion's or a rat's. Whereas they presumably can have emotional responses only to real, physical objects, our emotions, like our beliefs, may be about objects that are observed or unobservable, physical or mental, real or imagined (Elster 1999): 'If we had taken the left turn instead of the right we would be home by now'; 'I am an evil person for wishing him harm'; 'Oz must be beautiful'; 'I am afraid of dying'; 'Perhaps my success is responsible for your failure'. Furthermore, need,

---

[2] Perhaps it is because of the way the emotions work neurologically that it takes longer to shake off an emotion than a belief; or perhaps it because emotions are so much more complexly embedded in who one is.

[3] In a study done at Stanford, subjects were shown three different sorts of pictures: one sort was presumed to be emotionally neutral; the second showed 'negative' scenes, likely to arouse anger or stress of some sort (a picture of a mutilated baby, or people sobbing); the third was positive. Subjects were asked to try to think of an interpretation of a negative scene that would give it a more positive valence. As measured both by their subjective feelings and by functional imaging of the brain, they were successful (Gabrieli 2004).

wish, and emotion often inspire in us flights of imagination, as they probably do not in other animals, imaginative flights that in turn engender other emotions, and those complex mental structures we call fantasies. Perhaps it is because our carings are more complex than theirs that other animals wonder at us as the creatures who have lost our 'healthy animal reason'. Any adequate theory of the emotions must allow for some continuity between human and other creatures, and also for some enormous gaps.

Emphasizing the continuum, Darwin addressed the behavioral manifestations of emotions. But not all emotions have an outward show. Even if they did, describing it would tell us little about what an emotion is. This is the question addressed by the introspectionist psychologists Wundt and Titchner. The study of an emotion, they held, should consist in a systematic phenomenological description of one's state of consciousness during the experience of an emotion. Darwin told us how an emotion looks, the introspectionists how it feels.

James argued that the introspectionists left out the body, and he was equally critical of the 'classical' views of Locke and Hume for their 'atomistic' or 'building-block' view of mental life. Locke assumed there are primary states of mind that consist in simple sensations, themselves of two kinds: sensations of external objects and sensations of 'internal' things such as pleasure and pain. Sensations of sight, sound, smell, and so on belong to the former; basic emotions to the latter (Deigh 2001). Locke and Hume as well thought that these individual units of thought recur in different combinations and configurations to make the emotions in all their great variety.[4]

But our emotions and sensations are no more made up of atoms of sensation than rivers are made up of individual drops of water, James insisted. Just as one cannot step into the same river twice, so a sensation is also an unrepeatable experience, part of a stream of consciousness. Or, to change the metaphor, every feeling or emotion is embedded in an unduplicable life narrative. Tear Emma Bovary's disappointment, Ivan Karamazov's secret sense of guilt, from its narrative context, and 'the feeling' vanishes. 'The trouble with the emotions in psychology', James (1961: 242) writes, 'is that they are regarded too much as absolutely individual things . . .'

---

[4] Hume distinguished between sensations, or *impressions*, and *ideas*, which he held to differ from sensations only in vivacity.

The emotions are infinitely diverse, varying both with their contexts and with the objects that cause them. Spinoza (1963: 123) writes:

The pleasure which arises from the object, e.g. A, involves the nature of the object A, and the pleasure which arises from the object B involves the nature of that object B: and therefore these two pleasures are of different nature because they arise from causes of different nature. Thus also the emotion of sadness which arises from one object is different in nature from the sadness which arises from another cause . . .

James's own theory of the emotions is perverse, though it remains influential. James and the common view agree in thinking that emotions have a causal role in our explanations of behavior. According to the common view, the causal direction goes from the mental registration of some fact to the mental state we call the emotion, then from the emotion to the bodily expression, either in the form of blushing, tears, increased heart rate, or of voluntary action. James argues that this has things backwards. The causal direction is not from mind to body, but from body to mind: something causes us to blush, grow pale, tingle; then, if and when we become aware of this physiological state, we experience embarrassment, excitement, fear.

James is not necessarily denying that beliefs and desires have a role to play. Perhaps he would agree that in explaining Maria's anger we might begin by saying that she has seen or heard you do something she takes to be an insult. But, since this might happen without her experiencing an emotion, our quarry has escaped: 'Without the bodily states following on the perception, the latter would be purely cognitive in form, pale, colorless, destitute of emotional warmth' (James 1961: 243). On James's view, there is no emotion without physiological arousal, and feeling just is the perception of the arousal. We may correctly infer from someone's weeping that he is sad, not because sad thoughts are often expressed in weeping but because weeping often causes sadness.

James is right to insist that, for all their cognitive complexity, emotions are never merely cognitive constructions: this leaves out *feelings*. But emotions are not always felt; and feelings cannot always consist, as James says, of either perceptions of bodily arousal, or bodily arousal itself. For one thing, even when there is such arousal, there is often nothing in the *subjective* experience of it to distinguish one emotion from another. The more we attempt to isolate a feeling of fear from its psychological context, the less difference we are able to perceive between fear, for example, and any other kind of arousal. For another, often there is no perceived bodily arousal at all. Emotions are not merely cognitions; but neither are they cognitions plus something else.

Emotion as a Total Orientation to the World

James speaks of feeling as a perception of something inner. What is perceived, he says, is the subjective, emotional state, or disposition. So also Solms and Turnbull (2002: 106–7):

Only *you* can feel your emotions. This also applies to consciousness in general…but it applies to emotion in a special way. It is not only the *perception* of emotion that is subjective. *What* emotion perceives is subjective too. What you perceive when you feel an emotion is your *own subjective experience* of an event—not the event itself.

And even LeDoux (1996: 268)

My idea about the nature of conscious emotional experiences, emotional feelings, is incredibly simple. It is that a subjective emotional experience, like the feeling of being afraid, results when we become consciously aware that an emotion system of the brain, like the defense system, is active.

Of course, both the feeling and the emotion are subjective; but this does not mean that *what* is perceived is some 'inner', subjective event. That may be the case, as when I am anxiously aware of wishing harm to someone I love. But the perception, as in LeDoux's own example (see chapter 1), may be of the snake, or the angry expression on the father's face, or *that* someone is attempting to shame us. Through my own emotional reverberations I pick up the contempt or the fear in someone's voice, interpreting it, of course, in my own terms.

As a way of recovering from the inward focus of James and Solms, consider not the paradigmatic emotions and feelings—anger, fear, disgust—but the sort of feeling that in a trained and talented musician informs the music he is playing. 'Play it with feeling', the teacher says, meaning: your instruments (your dancer's body, your singer's voice, your pianist's hands) are ready; now relax, be alive to what is going on in the music, and in your fellow artists. Feeling is both part of what we use to 'get' the music or the words, and what we express when we do.[5]

We have rejected the ideas that an emotion is nothing but a cognitive configuration, and also that, cognitive or not, it must be marked by physiological arousal. Can we come closer to saying what an emotion is? One way to approach this is to ask, with Richard Wollheim: What are the respective roles in the mind of desire, belief, and emotion? Belief, he answers, provides the creature with a picture of the world it inhabits. Not just any picture, but one depicting the world more or less as it is. Desire provides the creature with ends, things at which to aim. Now, Wollheim (1995: 15) continues, 'the stage is set for the emotions. The role of emotion is to provide the creature . . . with an *orientation*, or an *attitude to the world*. If belief maps the world, and desire targets it, emotion tints or colours it: it enlivens it or darkens it, as the case may be.' Moran (1998: 181) similarly claims that, in comparison to belief, 'an emotional attitude constitutes something closer to a total orientation of the self, the inhabiting of a particular perspective'. Of all the psychological attitudes, we might then say that an emotion most identifies *what it is like* to be this particular person, taking in the world from this particular point of view.

It is an interesting grammatical fact that we speak both of knowing *what* we feel, and *how*, whereas there is no obvious use for 'I know how I believe . . .' or 'I know how I intend . . .'. Grammar suits the fact that, while beliefs and intentions are specific, typically articulable in propositions, emotions are total orientations, perhaps surfacing in feeling, or remaining latent as dispositions, like the framing attitudes that I spoke of in 'The Anxious Animal'. They are not transparent to the world, nor are they representations of it, but determinants of, background conditions for, our perceptual dispositions.

As orientations toward the world, emotions have intentionality. A feeling of melancholy, or joy, is *about* the world, the world conceived in a particular way, *as* empty, *as* full of promise, or *as* sad. An emotion is also intentional if it takes a proposition as its object: 'I feel ashamed *that* I want to embarrass you', 'proud that you have been so successful (or, for short, proud *of* your success)'. Yet, even when there is a propositional object, to construe the emotion simply as an attitude toward a

[5] I am not the first to notice that music is perhaps the best image we have of the life of feeling. Think of cadence, dynamics, harmonic resolution, tempo, rhythm, and so on.

proposition would slight the subjective, first-person, narrative, phenomenal character of an emotion, how it *feels* to be disposed toward the world, or a part of it, in an angry or a sad or a jealous way. 'The glass that is half full' and 'the glass that is half empty' describe the same glass; but the two perceptions carry a different emotional quality.

The presence of intentionality distinguishes emotions from the kinds of feelings that are bodily pain; the peculiar nature of their intentionality, and the fact that sometimes it is absent altogether, distinguish emotions from beliefs and desires. We might call the intentionality peculiar to the emotions as a *feeling toward*, which is 'thinking of with feeling' (Goldie 2000: 20). *Feeling toward* is not something that an analysis of emotion can just tack on to the content of an attitude like belief or desire; for the content of a feeling would not be what it is unless it were being experienced. The concept of feeling is irreducible, I suggest, and in that respect stands on a par with belief and desire.

Emotions and Communication

If emotions are peculiarly private or subjective states, that are also social in important ways. We are equipped from the beginning to communicate with each other, and emotions are our first messages. Paul Ekman's affect program theory makes this point.

The affect programs correspond roughly to the folk-psychological concepts of surprise, anger, fear, sadness, joy, and disgust, the emotions Ekman calls 'basic'.[6] They are stereotyped responses involving different bodily systems. Ekman discovered that, universally, these emotions are expressed by the same facial expressions, and that they are recognized cross-culturally. From this basic vocabulary of affects that we share with others, each of us develops one that is increasingly nuanced and complex, a development that itself happens in part through our interpersonal engagements.

Something like this process of emotional learning is, I believe, what Ronald de Sousa (1987: 45) means in saying that every person's emotional responses are a function of something he calls paradigm scenarios, 'little dramas in which our natural capacities for emotion

---

[6] See Paul Griffiths (1997) for a discussion of the strengths and weaknesses of affect program theory.

response were first enlisted'. De Sousa wants to grant that our emotional lives acquire complexity without resorting to the theory of emotional building blocks targeted by James. De Sousa (1987: 182) writes:

We are made familiar with the vocabulary of emotions by association with *paradigm scenarios*. These are drawn first from our daily life as small children and later reinforced by the stories, art, and culture, to which we are exposed. Paradigm scenarios involve two aspects: first, a situation type that provides the characteristic *objects* of the specific emotion-type . . . And second, a set of characteristic or 'normal' responses to the situation, where normality is first a biological matter, then very quickly becomes a cultural one.

As an example of the latter de Sousa gives the smiling response, a capacity for which is apparently inborn and that has no intentionality for the first few weeks: according to Daniel Stern's research, at first the baby smiles without any intention to communicate. But between six weeks and three months the infant begins to use the smile to get a response (Stern 1985). More and more the smile acquires meaning, and specific meanings that are determined by the context of specific relationships.

Our emotions increasingly become specific to us. Yet, even so, they remain to some extent communicable to others, and open to public appraisal. As friends, moralists, analysts, we sometimes feel that another's emotions are too strong for the occasion, or misplaced, or that she lacks an emotion it would be appropriate for her to have. Emotion fails her, we perhaps think, because she does not see, or will not see, the harm she has done, or that has been done to her; or because something inhibits her response.

But these are 'subjective' value judgments, one may object. Who is to say which feeling is appropriate to what situation, and when? It can seem as if asking 'subjective' or 'objective' about any value judgment is asking where the property in question is. Out there or in here? But it is not clear that this is a real question. Instead let us ask: is there room for dialogue, for amendment and correction of one's view? Yes, to the extent that we can argue a value judgment along rational lines. By pointing out details and features of a situation or object that I might have missed, or neglected, you may bring me to see and to feel for the first time the injustice in an act, the humor in a movie, the shamefulness of what I have done. Often this happens through the same sort of dialogue that, as I claimed earlier, expands our emotional repertoire; and insofar as a statement attributing a quality to a thing can be rationally defended, interpersonally argued, it is, in an important sense of the word, objective.

We are tempted to think of the emotions as belonging so entirely to our 'inner' lives that communication plays no role in shaping them. But this confuses 'inner' with 'incommunicable', and subjectivity with isolation. We first learn to discriminate those characteristics of a situation that make it an occasion for feeling pride, or shame versus guilt, or envy versus jealousy, through our intercourse with others. And since such discriminations enter into the very constitution of the emotions they too are sensitive to what I will call conversation. Clarifying what we feel is often a matter not just of putting new words to experiences that we already have, but of experiencing something new. For example: a particular feeling that I might have called 'my Sunday morning sadness' is now elaborated and refined through my reading of a Wallace Stevens poem. 'It' is no longer just the feeling that it was; neither is it something entirely new. We have difficulty talking about this in part, I think, because, as James pointed out, we tend to think of feelings as particular things, rather than as *ways in which* sequences of an ongoing journey are experienced.

Emotions are the register of what we care about. We have emotions because we *care* what happens to us, and care about things in the world as they relate to our vital interests. Nor would a care-less creature be rational in any sense that matters to us. Caring is implicit in all the emotions: if we did not care about what we do, about how people treat us, about who we are and about things and people in the world, we would not feel anger, fear, anxiety, pride, or envy, or anything else.

There is an obvious if often neglected fact about caring: the things we care about are things beyond our control, things on which our flourishing depends; our carings are concerned with things that come by surprise, that can be harmed and taken away from us, that grant or withhold gratification.[7] Deeply enmeshed in other mental states and dispositions as we ourselves are enmeshed in the external world, our emotions express our vulnerability to the ever-changing world around and within us. (From this point of view also it seems that Harry Frankfurt's idea that wholehearted caring depends on nothing outside

---

[7] This is a point well made by Robert Gordon (1987) and Martha Nussbaum (2001).

oneself cannot be right). The only creatures who are aware of their vulnerability, as we are in feeling fear, envy, shame, awe, or gratitude, we are also the only ones who wish to transcend it, the only ones to harbor fantasies of omnipotence or omniscience, to attempt to deny and cover over a painful sense of nakedness in the world. We are born to a world not of our making, and we become believing, desiring, impassioned creatures only through our relations with other such creatures, relations over which in the beginning we have no control. Long before Freud, Spinoza held that accepting our dependency on things outside ourselves is the key to emotional well-being.

Elster (1999: 403) eloquently remarks: 'Emotions matter because if we didn't have them, nothing else would matter.' Turn it around: emotion is how mattering shows up; the emotions help us know what matters to us, and sometimes why. They call into question a certain picture of reason itself, reason as cold, unmotivated, at a distance from the world, detached from the body, of objectivity as a stance bereft of feeling.

A consensus has been growing in psychoanalytic theory that places emotion, rather than 'drive', at the heart of a theory of motivation.[8] This emerging theory accommodates the fact that the child does not come equipped with a fixed repertoire of motives; it helps us understand both the flexibility and the fixity of human motivation; and, most important, it sees the individual as embedded in the world, becoming what she is only through interactions with other persons and things beyond her own skin.

---

[8] On this point see Westen (1997).

Self-Knowledge and Self-Discovery

Men are only free when they are doing what the deepest self likes.
And there is getting down to the deepest self. It takes some diving.

(D. H. Lawrence, *Studies in Classic American Literature*)

A true knowledge of good and evil cannot restrain any emotion in
so far as the knowledge is true, but only in so far as it is considered
as an emotion.

(Spinoza, *The Ethics*)

Self-knowledge is supposed to be transforming. Yet ordinarily, knowledge *by itself* has no effect on the object known. How can it, then,
when the object is one's self? What sort of knowledge is this? And what
sort of thing is it that is known?

In this chapter I take up first-person authority and the difficulties it
raises; then 'the ocular view' of self-knowledge and an alternative
account; finally, self-knowledge with regard to beliefs and to emotions.
Self-discovery often requires, I say, a dialectic between the first-person
and the third-person points of view in relation to one's self.

First-Person Authority

There are many things we can know about other persons. I know, or
think I do, that you are shorter than me, walk with splayed feet, live in
the Bronx. These sorts of characteristics you and I share with other
species, some characteristics even with inanimate objects.

But other characteristics define us as members of that particular
species that thinks, does things for reasons, and is animated by emotions

as complex as guilt and pride. I know, for example, or think I do, that you are gentle by temperament and fear being ignored at the same time as you are embarrassed by praise. I interpret what you do as expressing malice or generosity, or what you say as indicating that you believe it is raining outside, or I infer from your behavior that you are not going to invite me to your party. These are attributes of you that I discern from a third-person or 'objective' point of view; but they are ascribable only to persons, agents, subjects, who themselves have a first-person point of view.

So a view of you that is 'objective' in this sense must not be mistaken for a view that 'reduces' you to a mere, or merely physical, object, a point on which I insisted earlier. The important point about knowledge gained from this third-person point of view is that it is based on evidence. I can have such knowledge about myself: I can know that I— or someone I refer to as 'I'—have short hair, was born in Chicago, am named 'Marcia', have just uttered the words 'I hope you will understand me', am disposed to impatience.

I can also know that I am now thinking about going to the symphony, or that I am hungry, or that in my mind's eye I am picturing you when you were 12. But, in contrast to third-person knowledge of myself, I know these things in the absence of evidence, or 'immediately': *I just know*. We call this knowledge of oneself from the position of the first person. We grant it authority in the following sense: in an ordinary and unproblematic situation you might ask me why I believe it is raining outside (you see no rain on the windows), but you will not ask how I know this is what I believe. You presume that I do know, and without having to consult anything beyond myself.

Freud, by the way, did not deny first-person authority. To be sure he thought we know our own minds less well than we think we do, but he took his therapeutic task in any given case to be widening the authority with which a patient can speak for herself. Where now I insist I believe in my father's integrity, for example, or that his failure is to some extent my fault, or that I am a total incompetent in the world, I may be moved to question these beliefs, and finally to acknowledge a more ambiguous or even radically different belief from the one I first professed.

There are basic challenges to a philosophic position that maintains first-person authority. We must resolve the apparent contradictions between the private and the public, the inner and the outer. We must privilege my knowledge of myself, while granting the publicity of what I know; for, if this is knowledge in anything like the standard sense, then what is known must be objectively knowable, that is, by others as well as by myself. We must provide for our common-sense distinction between self-apprehensions that can be said to be illusory and clear-eyed, self-knowledgeable and self-deceptive. We must maintain a sense of privacy that is compatible with human connectedness, since, without the latter, I have argued, there is no mind. And, finally, we must explain how, if it is not based on evidence, my knowing my own mind can be a form of empirical knowledge at all.

To the last question, the so-called ocular model, which many people still find persuasive, was for a long time the best answer going: think of mental contents as resembling things in the world, but unlike them in that they are available only to the inner eye. (Kant called it 'the inner sense'.) I can be mistaken about who the man is walking down the street, whether it is a man, what he is wearing, and so on, but I cannot be mistaken about what I think I see, what I *see* with my mind's eye. On this model the distinction between how things *are* and how things appear drops out, such that mental content all by itself amounts to a way of having knowledge.

The ocular model explains first-person authority as deriving from the purported facts that mental contents are available only to the mind whose contents they are, and that they are self-identifying. To know that the man crossing the street is my friend Bruce, I must re-cognize him, recognize him *as* Bruce; just this gap between Bruce-in-the-world and my representation of Bruce makes room for error. But, it can seem, my mind's eye needs nothing beyond itself and its own moment. The phenomenological content of the thought alone tells me that it is about Bruce. Hence the immediacy and the supposed certainty of this sort of self-knowledge.

The problems with this view are well rehearsed.

1. Mental content is not, and cannot be, self-identifying. This is a point that has been familiar since Wittgenstein, Richard Moran writes, 'and was part of his original case against the perceptual model. And when he asks, "How do I know that I am imagining King's College on fire, and not another one just like it?" his point is not to suggest any

doubt about what he is imagining, but to point out that "visual" properties do not determine content or one's knowledge of it' (Moran 2001: 16). The content of a belief, say that the Second World War ended in 1945, is constituted by a multitude of inferential commitments about related matters, for example, about wars in general and the Second World War in particular, a view I referred to earlier in this book as 'mental holism'. To think that you can read off the content of a belief by 'looking' at it is like thinking you can read off the referent of a Rembrandt self-portrait just by looking at its surface. The surface tells you many things, but it does not give you the painting's internationality.

2. Clearly we do make mistakes about our own minds. We deceive ourselves; we discover, like Socrates' interlocutors, that we do not really understand what we are saying; we ride an emotional wave without knowing what it is.

3. Sometimes, as the ocular view maintains, we have a mental picture or image, but more often we do not; rather, we find out what we are thinking in the very act of thinking it. The ocular model fails to capture just the sort of self-discovery that defines psychoanalytic therapy. That is by no means its only site, but it provides a paradigm in envisioning self-discovery as a temporal process that often takes place in an interpersonal relationship structured by a shared physical space. In this relationship one is seen and identified with from the outside; one sees oneself from and identifies with the position of the other. In short, the ocular view is untrue to the very thing on which it relies: the phenomenology of the self-knower's experience.

4. Who, on the ocular view, is the observer of the mental contents? And what is the relationship between observer and observed? Hume asks us to think of the mind as a theater in which ideas parade across an inner stage. But where is the thinker? In the audience? On the stage? Is she somehow independent of her thoughts? To say any of these things would lose touch with the phenomenon of first-person authority altogether.

Thus the ocular view does not sufficiently capture just how 'personal' first-person knowledge is. This is Richard Moran's elegant point: the model posits 'objects' in the form of percepts or mental pictures that are privileged because they are 'visible' only on one's own inner stage; but pictures are the sorts of things that are in principle available to others.[1] Saying that I and only I can see them does not do justice to the fact that my thoughts are deeply embedded in my character, emotions, and history. The view ignores the fact that the first-person perspective of any one person is part of what constitutes that person as that particular person; it gives us subjectivity without a subject and that absolutely excludes others rather than a subjectivity that is implicit in what it is to be a person, a person separate from others, but not closed off.

5. Finally, if the knowledge that we have of our own minds can be said to be genuinely *knowledge*, its claims must be sensitive to both truth and falsity. Rather than a wrinkle to be smoothed away, the possibility of error is essential to first-person authority. And, rather than ruling out the knowledge of other minds, first-person authority demands that at least some aspects of the mind be knowable from a third-person point of view.

Wittgenstein (1972) pointed the way to a reconception of first-person authority that accommodates these ideas. He imagines the following dialogue: ' "I don't know if this is a hand" [the Cartesian skeptic]. But do you know what the word "hand" means?' (p. 39). 'If I wanted to doubt whether this was my hand, how could I avoid doubting whether the word "hand" had any meaning?' (p. 48). And again: 'If I don't know *that*, how do I know that my words mean what I believe they mean?' (p. 66). Wittgenstein is saying that sometimes my knowing what I believe is a matter of knowing what I *mean* by what I say, just as my knowing what you believe is sometimes knowing what you mean. The difference is that I know what you mean only through inference: I begin with some knowledge of your language, and I go on to fill in what you mean not only from the words of a single sentence alone, say, 'Here's a human hand', but also from the context of your saying it, your behavior, and from my understanding of what other things you believe and feel. My knowing what I mean, on the other hand, requires no such inference.

But it does require a context. Though I need not be aware of them, there are conditions that have to be in place before I can know what

[1] My views in this chapter are deeply indebted to Richard Moran (2001). There are two chief differences between our treatments of self-knowledge. I discuss: (1) knowing one's own emotions; and (2) what I call a dialectic in self-discovery between the first-person and the third-person perspective on one's self.

I mean, even use the first-person pronoun intelligibly. We might then recast the question about first-person authority as asking: How do we become creatures who are able to invest our words and gestures with meaning? Davidson answers with the 'triangulation' argument I presented in Chapter 4. He asks us to consider the following: 'Someone who is consciously teaching a beginner the use of a word may think of herself as simply passing on a meaning that is already attached to the word. But from the learner's point of view, the word—the sound—is being *endowed* with a meaning' (Davidson 2001: 14).

The point is that the learner is investing a sound with meaning and not just recognizing a meaning that is already there, let alone there, as Barry Smith (2003) puts it, 'on the surface of other people's meaningful speech'. Elaborating Davidson's position, Barry Smith writes:

For a speaker or language learner to take a word to mean something it takes more than just the ability to utter the word. Moreover, the word's meaning something to me is not constituted solely by my taking it to mean something... But if it is not the seeming impression of meaning that gives the word a meaning for me, why does knowing that it means such and such seem to require little more from me than my taking it to mean such and such? The answer is that it is only when certain further conditions are met that my taking the word to mean such and such will coincide what it means... The further conditions involve links to others from whom I learned the word. (Smith 2003).

Perhaps we never know fully what we mean. We are like the child parroting words he does not yet understand; or the person on the brink of a thought or an intuition; or a poet, struck by an isolated phrase that later emerges as a poem; or a patient in analysis saying 'I have the feeling that I'm sort of trying to prove to you I'm right, but I'm really not sure if that is what I am doing'; or someone like Euthyphro, who discovers through Socrates' relentless examination that he has not begun to consider the implications of something he thinks he believes.

But might it be that I never know, never even begin to know? The point of Davidson's arguments on the connection between knowing what one means and knowing one's own mind is that total ignorance of this sort is inconceivable. If you discovered about someone you had taken to be a person that he did not know what he meant by *any* of his words, then in his mouth they would not be words. You would have no reason for thinking he ever meant anything, had a mind at all. First-person authority is a constitutive feature of being a person, an agent: you can challenge my authority on a particular occasion, but you cannot, without denying my status as a person, challenge my authority in general. Recognizing another as having such authority is recognizing him as a creature with whom, in principle, we can engage in dialogue.

We are creatures who have an 'outside' and an 'inside', both of which are mediated through the external world. Sometimes it is assumed that we can treat them in isolation from each other, or omit one aspect altogether. But we see that, on the contrary, our account of self-knowledge must recognize the ways in which the external world, including relationships with others, is part of the fabric of the inner world, as one's first-person experience provides the only approach to one's knowledge of the external world. This is self-evident; yet, because of the ways in which experience itself is partly constituted by memory, discipline, language, and interplay between organism and surrounding world, it is more problematic than it first appears.

We have resolved the seeming contradictions between the subject-ivity demanded by *self*-knowledge and the publicity demanded by self-*knowledge*, in distinguishing *what* I know from *how* I know it. That I am greedy, or generous, or have just made a malicious remark, is knowable by both of us; but unique to me are some of the ways in which I know it.

Knowing what I Believe

Let me now address one's own mind in more detail. I begin with knowing what I believe, for belief brings into focus once again the relations between mind and world.

Gareth Evans has argued that, if I am in a position to assert that p, then I am also in a position to say 'I believe that p' (Evans 1982). From there to knowing I believe that p is not an additional step, but comes with knowing how to make an assertion. Suppose I now come to question whether I believe that p. What I must do is check the truth of p. That is, determining what I believe is often not a matter of looking inward, but outward, toward that part of the world that my belief is about. Evans calls this feature of belief 'transparency'.

Where the belief is simple, say a straightforward perceptual belief, transparency is simple; it is more complex as the belief itself becomes more complicated. Take my earlier example: I am praising my father's integrity, and you, reminding me of my having hesitantly told you a week ago about his laundered Swiss bank accounts, ask skeptically: 'Are you sure you believe he had integrity?' Now my checking on what I believe is going to be more difficult, partly because belief here is so colored by pain and pleasure. I turn inward. I say, perhaps, 'Yes, I did say that. But I still want to insist that he was a man of honor. I guess I am in some conflict about this.' Perhaps I go on to reflect.

When beliefs are affectively complex in this way, 'transparency' may demand virtues that are equally complex. Where transparency has been lost, restoring it requires a new orientation of the believer to reality.

Whatever the content, I can know what I believer only if I acknow-ledge in general, and in this particular case, what holding a belief commits me to: fidelity to what I see; a readiness to appraise and reap-praise the belief in the light of new considerations and evidence; and the integrity to sort this belief with others of my beliefs. I think this is what Moran means in calling knowing what one believes a matter of *avowal*. Merely believing does not make these commitments. But knowing what I believe, or avowing my belief, does.

Someone who, willfully or otherwise, does not attend to what is going on outside or inside of her, or whose focus is highly restricted by anxiety, or strong passion, is not, on those occasions, in a good position to know either her own mind or the world. We can know what we believe in general, yet fail to be rational believers on particular occa-sions, or with regard to certain kinds of things; and it is generally, if not always, the emotions, in particular those Spinoza calls passions, that lead us astray.

Knowing what I Feel

Recall from the opening chapter LeDoux's basic points about emotional memory.

1. The emotional system is in charge of appraising the meaning of a stimulus in terms of one's own welfare, or the welfare of some-thing or someone one cares about.

2. Much of this appraisal goes on beneath conscious awareness, such that the organism can evaluate the emotional meaning of an event as 'good' or 'bad' before it knows just what the event is and what is bad about it.

3. The appraisals may be automatic, unconscious, non-verbal, implicit, and non-declarative; but for creatures capable of propositional thought they can also be, at some point in the emotional process, declarative, conscious, and cognitively laden.

4. Often something makes an emotional impact that bypasses cognition entirely.

Damasio (1994) speaks of emotion as a combination of a mental evaluative process and a dispositional response to that process. According to his 'somatic-marker' hypothesis, emotions are an essential part of practical reason giving the creature a sense of how the world relates to its goals and projects. Something more than a merely intellectual rehearsal of possible outcomes enters our deliberations about what to do, and this something more is feelings. Somatic markers are feelings generated by what Damasio calls secondary emotions, the ones that learning has connected, via the high road LeDoux describes, to certain situations. Somatic markers assist the reasoning process by highlighting some options as dangerous, others as favorable. If in the past an alternative similar to the one we are now considering had been connected with something 'bad', then, however fleetingly, we may experience an unpleasant gut feeling, which functions like a signal of anxiety, quickly alerting us to danger. This is the wisdom in the advice to trust out feelings. But if we also recall, from Chapter 1, the distinctions between implicit and explicit memory, and the different ways in which memories can be organized, we see that feelings can also be misleading. Knowing one's own emotional state is often a task of enormous complexity.

Knowing what one feels is sometimes a matter of painfully acknowledging what one knows against the pressure of a wish not to know; put the other way around: where knowing is acknowledging, feeling is a necessary part of believing. A person who was capable of believing that his actions are blameworthy, for example, but incapable of feeling shame or guilt, would be as estranged from himself as someone who was able only to predict rather than to decide what he would do, or state what he believes as conclusions from evidence. Such a person would not count as an agent. It is not clear that we would even credit him with the beliefs he espouses.

In a vignette that Moran takes from a novel by Kingsley Amis, a man sneaks home to his wife after a secret escapade with a colleague. The man guiltily describes himself to himself as feeling a tremendous 'rakehell' 'and not liking myself much for it, and feeling rather a good chap for not liking myself much for it, and not liking myself at all for feeling a rather good chap' (Moran 2001: 174–5). Clearly this self-reflexive process could go on *ad infinitum*. Something has gone wrong. But what? Someone else can sensibly commend the man for feeling ashamed. Why can he not sensibly commend himself?

On Moran's subtle analysis, the commendation is warranted only if the man still feels ashamed, since there is nothing laudatory about having felt ashamed in the past. Nor would there be anything to laud now if he no longer thought his behavior shameful. So where is the room for commendation? Only in the gap between a 'straight' belief that he did something shameful, and the corresponding emotional attitude of feeling ashamed. If such a gap existed, then it might be possible for him to continue to believe that he did something shameful, while now feeling not ashamed but pleased with himself.

But the idea of such a gap raises another problem: Is the mere belief alone, without the felt acknowledgment—that is, the feeling of shame—sufficient to warrant the commendation? Moran (2001: 182) writes: 'what matters to the success or legitimacy of the expressive interpretation, it seems, is the shame itself: how it orients the person, the fact that it is something hard to undergo, and what *experiencing* it implies about the quality of the person's attitude toward what he did as well as his attitude toward the future.' In feeling himself a good chap for feeling ashamed, the man effectively admits that he is not ashamed. In which case there is no ground for praise. *One form of knowing what one feels consists in acknowledging it.*

Of course one can acknowledge feeling only what one does in fact feel. And here self-knowledge encounters another problem: unlike beliefs and intentions, feelings can be not merely hidden and denied, but strangled at the root. Or they can, on the contrary, be developed, played out, nourished, expressed. We repress and disavow both beliefs and affects; but only feelings do we 'inhibit', 'go with', 'turn off'; only feelings flow, catch us up, flood and overwhelm us. On Freud's earliest model of pathology, therapy consists in releasing affect that has been damned up. It is true that such damning-up happens, and that this is a primary way in which a human life gets blocked. These are important metaphors that Freud for a while took literally. What do the metaphors convey? That emotion is often inchoate, inarticulate, sometimes because something is working against its expression, sometimes because expression requires time, training, work.

Articulating a feeling may be a matter of letting it grow, or expressing it, by which I do not mean acting it out, as I express my anger in striking you, or my impatience in tapping my foot. Nor do I have in mind a relation between outward form and inner impulse, as the baby's scowl expresses anger, or its smile contentment. I mean expression as something an agent *does*, say in working with words, or clay, or sounds; or in *working through* a revelatory or transforming experience. Crying may not be expressive in this sense, but mourning is. In this sense, expression brings to the feeling an articulation it did not yet have: I discover what I (potentially) feel about that prancing bird in writing the haiku; about the loss of James in mourning him. I may discover something about who I am in writing a memoir that forces me to take a stance, create a voice.

Dewey writes that, in making a work of art, physical materials must be altered. So also the 'inner' elements, and, most important, the emotions. This way of putting it misleadingly suggests that there are two different operations, but in fact there is only one; for ordering the material, or putting something into words, is also an ordering of the raw, unformed emotion. So also when we are talking together, or trying to work something out between us. An irritated person is moved to do something. He can enact the irritation directly. But he can also express it indirectly, perhaps remembering that a certain physical activity helps when he is feeling this way. 'As he puts objects in order his emotion is ordered . . .' and transformed (Dewey 1934: 74). *A second form of knowing what one feels consists in expressing it.*

Sometimes articulating the inarticulate is desperately hard. Sometimes easy. It depends on who one is and what skills are at her disposal. At the beginning of one of her many quick voyages to self-discovery, Emma Woodhouse is trying to talk Harriet out of her interest in Mr Knightly. Emma thinks she is doing this because Harriet will be hurt, since of course Mr Knightly cannot be interested in Harriet.

But she assures Emma that the interest is reciprocated. Austen (n. d.: 418) writes:

Emma's eyes were instantly withdrawn. A few minutes were sufficient for making her acquaintance with her own heart. A mind like hers, once opening to suspicion, made rapid progress. She touched, she admitted, she acknowledged the whole truth. Why was it so much worse that Harriet should be in love with Mr Knightly than with Frank Churchill? Why was the evil so dreadfully increased by Harriet's having some hope of a return? It darted through her with the speed of an arrow that Mr Knightly must marry no one but herself.

Emma expresses her feelings in the thought about Mr Knightly, and therein knows her heart. Compare this Emma with Flaubert's Emma Bovary:

This temperament, positive in the midst of its enthusiasms, which had loved the church for its flowers, the music for the romantic lyrics, and literature for its passion-inspiring stimulation, rebelled before the mysteries of faith in proportion to her growing irritation with the discipline, which was anti-pathetic to her nature. When her father came to take her from the convent, the sisters were not sorry to see her go.

Back home Emma amused herself at first by taking charge of the servants, then she began disliking the country and missed the convent. When Charles came to Les Berteaux for the first time, she felt quite disillusioned, having nothing more to learn, nothing more to feel.

But the uneasiness at a new role or perhaps the disturbance caused by the presence of this man, had been sufficient to make her believe that she finally felt that marvelous passion that until now had been like a huge pink-winged bird soaring through the splendor of poetic skies. She could not believe that the calm in which she was now living was the happiness of which she had dreamed. (Flaubert 1965: 59)

Perhaps, we are told, Emma feels 'uneasiness' over her new role, or 'disturbance' in the presence of this man. She believes she is feeling the transcendent passion of which she has read. Were she to be self-knowledgeable in this instance she would know that her longing for such a passion may be hindering her judgment. She would come to recognize that she cares for nothing and no one but herself, and that she is emotionally impoverished: her affective repertoire lacks the expansive emotions of affection, curiosity, love, gratitude, awe; it is limited to anger, resentment, envy, hatred, malice, longing, guilt unacknowledged.

No one could discover this on her own; and with what tact the teaching would have to be done. Emma is doomed. Self-discovery may not come easily, if at all, to one who has been emotionally starved; furthermore, privation itself motivates illusion and self-deception.

Comparing the two Emmas makes clear that character can predispose one to emotional wisdom or ignorance. Emma Bovary's emotional life is too impoverished at the beginning of her descent for her to be capable even of self-deception. When Lear's daughters tell each other that their father has known himself. But slenderly, they mean that he is too bent on power, too easily blinded by pride and arrogance, to be in a position to know himself on any particular occasion. Sometimes self-discovery, then, will come only with characterological change that has already been set in motion: not first, self-discovery, then change; but change, then discovery, and with it self-discovery.

Self-Understanding and the Passions

Spinoza distinguishes the emotions in general from the more particular emotions he calls passions, which include wrath, envy, jealousy, resentment, hate, shame, regret. The latter emotions are natural, but unchecked they tend to be destructive not only of persons but also of clarity of mind. (For example, in anger, envy, rage, and fear, I see not a whole person or a whole situation, but a caricature.) What determines the place of an emotion on this spectrum is how well it is understood. The passions are emotions of which one has only what Spinoza calls 'an inadequate idea'—that is, a misunderstanding. When we have an 'adequate idea' of an emotion, or an idea that is relatively so, its cause is a part of the content of what we are feeling. I am sad, and a part of my very feeling of sadness is the idea that Sandra has gone away. Her disappearance is the true cause of my feeling, and essential to what it is feel. To the degree that my idea that my idea is inadequate, I am sure neither of what I am feeling nor of what is causing me to feel it. We discussed the relation between the content and the cause of an emotion earlier (see Chapter 9).

The passions are destructive in yet another way in that they create inner conflict, and so generate self-deception. In fear, or rage, or envy, for example, I naturally wish to harm the one who causes me pain, and feel pleasure when I do. But, at the same time, I am by nature equally inclined in every instance to be affected by an emotion like that I perceive in another. (When the other is experiencing pain this response is called 'compassion'.) Thus, while harming someone who threatens me or whom I envy is pleasurable, it also pains me. This conflict then induces me to blind myself to what I do, to the pain of the other, and to my own agency. (As in Freud, for Spinoza, conflict and defense against conflict shape the basic drama of the mind). Before I was merely confused; now I am both confused and self-estranged.

Take envy. Envy arises, Spinoza says, when we think someone enjoys something we do not have, or think we do not have, and believe it to be something only one person can possess. We are then motivated to wrest the envied good away from him, and feel pleasure when we succeed. And here begins the affective conflict and the self-deception just described.

Were I, on the contrary, to work towards an adequate idea of my envy in a given instance, I would, of course, know what I envy and why; I would also be aware of my beliefs that the envied good could be mine, and that its belonging to another prevents it from being mine, beliefs that, on reflection, I might find false; and I would further understand that envy is corrosive of my own well-being. Now I would be in position to assess my beliefs and to bring my experience to bear on the affect itself. Thus can we can tutor an emotion if and when we are able to be aware of it and comprehend its consequences—not the actual consequences that we can know only in the future, but those consequences that are implicit in the very description of the emotion, as self-divisiveness is implicit in envy.

Reason, which both cultivates the emotions and is itself enhanced through their education, requires, Spinoza tells us, that in addition to our having relatively adequate ideas of our emotions, we accept ourselves as what we are: a part of Nature, a vast system over which we have little control. So we are back to vulnerability, and its acknowledgment.

Does Spinoza put too much faith in reason? Yes, if we think of reason as a faculty distinct from will and desire. But this Cartesian conception of reason as passive and unmotivated is one of Spinoza's targets. Nietzsche wonderfully spoke of Spinoza's 'making knowledge the most powerful affect' (quoted in Curley 1998: 128). A stunning idea! And so with knowledge as we come to understand it in the light of psychoanalysis. We can say that the psychoanalytic process heads toward self-knowledge, so long as we understand this 'knowledge' to be both a new affective state, and a new relation to external as well as internal reality.

Earlier I distinguished knowing oneself as an object in the world from knowing oneself as an 'I' from one's own first-person position. Sartre similarly distinguishes between a theoretical attitude toward oneself and the practical attitude of an agent. On the first, I explain or predict my behavior in the same way that I explain or predict yours: 'I have a stingy character because I grew up envious of my brother'; or 'I probably won't take the job because I'm just too fearful of change'. On the second, I decide, and I act.

By 'the vertigo of consciousness', Sartre (1960: 74) meant our uneasy awareness that the self of which we are aware as fully conscious believers, desirers, doers, is not something knowable and fixed, but a kind of spontaneity toward the world, an endless array of possibilities. On his diagnosis, we construe the self as a special kind of entity, behind and directing our various acts of consciousness, because we don't want to acknowledge that who and what we are is up to us. 'Perhaps,' he writes, 'the essential function of the Ego is not so much theoretical as practical . . . to mask from consciousness its very spontaneity' (1960: 81).

Sartre thinks that in taking the theoretical attitude I construe myself as something given rather than something I am continually making. And he holds that only the latter view is appropriate to the kind of creature that I am: free, responsible, a creature that can avow its beliefs and its intentions. It is true that both explaining and predicting my own behavior can elide the difference between an action, between something done for reasons, and a bit of unminded behavior, between my lighting the kindling and the kindling's catching fire. Explanation and prediction can serve to excuse rather than to reflect, to turn into a fixed fact about oneself something that by its nature is the outcome of evaluation, choice, and decision.

But the difference between the given and the made is not exclusive. Since we are creatures in the material world who can be seen and interpreted by others, and who also see and make interpretations from our first-person position, we might expect that self-discovery often consists in a dialogue between the two points of view. Sometimes the objective stance is taken by oneself; sometimes by another person, who provides a perspective on myself from which I, perhaps see things about myself to which I may have been oblivious.

The person we describe as knowing herself has a good sense of her own character, capabilities, talents, limitations, and worldly situation. She has learned how she tends to frame the world, what assumptions and affects she brings to her perceptions. Emma Bovary needs to discover that she experiences the world against a horizon of unrealizable demand. Emotions are themselves both framed and framing, determining how the world is viewed. As I become more adept at observing myself, new observations of the world become possible; new observations then generate new feelings. Rather than discharge there is reflection: How am I thinking about the object of my feeling? How do I understand what I am feeling?

My opening questions were: What sort of knowing is it that can change the thing known? And what sort of thing is one's self such that it can be both subject of and object for one's discoveries? The first question addresses knowledge, the second, the self; but, because the knower is the known, the questions are separable only provisionally. Self-knowledge is puzzling in principle if one holds that the 'I' is a timeless, indivisible entity. It is puzzling if one thinks we have to choose between saying that either the human creature is a kind of object in the world to be known through observation, or a subject. The illusion would rather be to think that anything other than death can close the gap between who we are and who we might become.

APPENDIX

Knowledge, Consensus, and Uncertainty

My own beliefs are held with a skepticism which I never even hope to be quite rid of.

(T. S. Eliot)

The idea of knowledge has been a central theme in psychoanalysis from the beginning. We hear it in the claims that self-knowledge is a route to psychic health, and that psychoanalytic therapy puts us more in touch both with ourselves and with reality; again in psychoanalytic theories about the origins and the vicissitudes of thinking. It is agreed that part of the therapeutic enterprise is to make us better thinkers, explorers, knowers. Yet, with the idea of the unconscious, Freud gave us post-Cartesian reasons for skepticism about our ability to know anything at all. Contemporary clinicians have yet other epistemological anxieties: we are more alert than perhaps Freud was to the limitations imposed by our own culture, sex, and place in history; wary of assuming that the psychoanalyst occupies some privileged position from which to judge that the patient has things wrong; less confident that our own values are beyond challenge; rather, we now assume the psychoanalyst's observational stance is *within* an intersubjective field.

I want to address these concerns first with some general considerations about knowledge. Then I will turn to ones more specific to psychoanalysis.

A good place to begin is with Plato's dialogue the *Theaetetus*, not because it was the first systematic treatment of knowledge in Western philosophy, though it was, nor because philosophers have learned nothing about knowledge since then, but because Plato makes distinctions that philosophers continue to acknowledge and of which any epistemological theory has at least to be mindful. Plato set the major problems for epistemology down to our own time.

Socrates asks a young student named Theaetetus 'What is knowledge?' 'Knowledge is nothing but perception,' Theaetetus ventures (Plato 1973: 151 e5).

It is a maddeningly ambiguous answer, as under Socrates' tutelage we soon realize. One might begin to show its ambiguity to a contemporary audience by asking 'Is knowing that New York is the biggest city in the United States perceiving *that* it is?' What do I perceive when I have this knowledge? A view from an airplane will show me New York, but, by itself, it will not show me that New York is big, since that is a comparative concept, nor that it is the biggest city in the United States. And so on.

What do we mean by 'perceive'? A baby, a snake, and I can all perceive, in one sense of the word, the lily in the garden. This sort of perception requires nothing but sensory receptors. But presumably only I can see the lily *as* a lily, since that requires having the concept of a lily, and not just that concept, but many others, since, if I know about lilies, presumably I understand also such related concepts as flower, plant, growing thing, tree (which I will know a lily is not). *Seeing as* is a kind of seeing that locates the object perceived in a vast network of interlocking conceptual discriminations.

If one sees the lily *as* a lily, does one see *that* it is a lily? Presumably. And like *seeing as, seeing that* is a kind of seeing, a kind of perceiving, that neither snake nor baby can do. Seeing *that* something is the case is a propositional sort of seeing. When one sees *that p*, one recognizes or believes it to be the case *that p*. One can identify, and sometimes misidentify, what one is seeing as a lily.

The ambiguity in 'perception' is matched by an ambiguity in 'know'. In one sense of the word the baby 'knows' its mother, the dog its master's footsteps. Something like this sort of knowing is what Bion (1997) has in mind when he speaks of knowing as one of the three basic emotional experiences linking objects that are in relationship to each other. But there are things *about* the mother and the master that presumably neither the baby nor the dog knows. It is pretty clear that they have no knowledge of a propositional kind, knowledge that brings with it such psychological activities as doubting, questioning, arguing, seeing something from the point of view of another.

Believing that something is the case is not a merely sensory matter; believing is not the same as knowing; and knowing (the woman next door) is not the same as knowing *that* (the woman you just saw is the woman next door). Nor is either of these knowings the same as knowing *how*. Theaetetus was not making these distinctions, so he had not even begun to ask himself about the respective roles of sensation, cognition, and conception in what we call thinking, believing, and knowing.

It has always been tempting in epistemology to confuse the question, 'What do I know?' with the question 'How do I know it?' So the British Empiricists said that, since all knowledge is based on sensory experience, our own sense data are *what* we know. Some Idealists say that the world just is Idea—to which

Schopenhaur added, Will. But is it not rather the case that, unless I am blind or somehow grossly deceived, what I know, or perceive, from the deck of my house in Berkeley, for example, are the bay and the Golden Gate Bridge? My eyes and my particular visual experience are the answer to how I know in this case what is before me, but what I see are the bay and the bridge. That is what you see too, if you are not blind, or grossly deceived; though of course the bay and the bridge will look slightly different to each of us and will bring different associations to mind. *How* I know there is a bridge involves things going on in my sense organs, though not only these.

Socrates asks Theaetetus to clarify his statement that knowledge is nothing but perception. Perhaps Theaetetus has in mind something like the Protagorean view, Socrates suggests, that 'everything is, for me, the way it appears to me, and is, for you, the way it appears to you' (152a7). Theaetetus says this is what he had in mind. But can Theaetetus really mean that things *are* the way they appear to any person at any moment? This would lead us to flat-out contradictions. If the same object can appear *x* to me, not-*x* to you, even different to me myself at different moments, and if how things appear just is how they are, it would follow that the same object can *be* both *x* and not-*x*, the same proposition can *be* both false and true. What is wrong with this suggestion is that it undermines the very possibility of making sense; we would not be able ever to mean what we say. The law of non-contradiction is not a constraint imposed on thought from something beyond, but a condition of meaning. How could I understand any claim if all our claims were self-contradictory? Which is not to deny that we can have conflicted feelings, nor that we can believe that *x* is *a* from one point of view, and not-*a* from another. Socrates concludes that Theaetetus cannot mean that things *are* the way they seem to each person at any moment, but that people *think* the way things seem to them is the way they are. Susan Haack (1999: 13) makes the point this way: 'Although what is true is not relative to perspective, what is accepted as true is; although incompatible statements cannot be jointly true, incompatible claims are frequently made.' This is the distinction Theatetus slurs.

Let us start again. What is knowledge? We have mentioned one unproblematic condition: knowledge requires belief. If I know that *p*, I must at least believe that *p*. Belief is a subjective state, but of a special kind; for, unlike sensations of hot and cold, or moods of depression and elation, or feelings of anger and gratitude, belief, as Bernard Williams (1973: 148) has put it, 'aims at the true'. This means, for one thing, that a belief is by definition something that can be true or false, and that a creature who has the concept of belief knows this. It means, for another, that it is not possible to believe something that one also thinks, in the same part of one's mind, so to speak, is false; for to think that *p* is not true just is, in the standard case, not to believe it.

Again, there are, of course, aberrant cases: we often hold beliefs that we know in some sense are not rationally justified; one can know something—'in one's head', or 'in one part of one's mind'—yet not wholeheartedly believe it, know something consciously but unconsciously believe something incompatible with it. So the belief condition is more problematic than we thought. Still, though these aberrations call for qualifications on the theme of knowing and believing, they are not the standard case, without which we could not recognize an aberration for what it is.

Yet belief is not sufficient for knowledge, for one thing because I can have false beliefs, and a false belief is not knowledge: we sometimes discover that we only thought we knew. We were wrong in claiming to know that *p* because *p* turned out to be false. Wittgenstein (1972: 8e) asks us to consider whether the difference between belief and knowledge stems 'from the difference between the mental states of belief and knowledge'. That is, is knowledge, like belief, a subjective state, just more special in kind? Well, only creatures who are subjects can have knowledge. But knowledge is not subjective in the sense that your knowing that *p* is only in part up to you, or dependent on conditions 'internal' to you. You can think you know without its being the case that you do, for, if you genuinely know that *p*, things are as *p* says. This is where reality comes in. Knowledge is a condition of a particular, minded, partial, fallible, creature, that nevertheless connects him to the way things are. To say it connects him to the way things *really* are is redundant: we cannot do epistemology without running into metaphysics.

A second condition on knowledge, then, is that the belief be true. In the Middle Ages, scientists thought, on the basis of the best evidence then available, furthermore, that the earth was flat. They thought they knew this to be the case. We now say they *thought* they knew it. It may help to think of truth not as some ideal entity with a capital T, but rather as a property that some beliefs and sentences have. Language, including the concept of truth, is a human construct. This does not imply, however, that truth and reality are also human constructs, whatever that would mean. Nor need it be the case that the concept of truth varies from culture to culture, though of course the particular beliefs we hold true do vary, so also what we consider reliable evidence. To assess the truth of an utterance you have to know what it means to this particular speaker (believer), speaking this particular language. You cannot know if the sentence 'New York is big' is true unless you understand it, and know also the relevant standard of size. But, once you know these things, you can assess the truth of the claim. And, if you decide that the sentence is true, you think New York is big.

So far, then, knowledge is true belief. Are belief and truth sufficient conditions? No, for a reason that has already emerged. Knowledge requires not only that one's belief be true, but also that the believer have good reasons for holding it, and that he holds it, at least in part, *because* of these reasons. If I hit on a true belief by accident—say it is a lucky guess (my bet at the Kentucky Derby pays off)—we would not call it knowledge. Or your true belief might be an illusion in Freud's sense (1927). For all we know, you may be, as you believe, in the hands of an all-powerful and all-loving God; perhaps there is even evidence to support this belief. But if *you* believe it *because* it relieves you of anxiety, then you do not *know* that it is true. Reasons for believing that take the form of wishes, or fears, or intra-psychic conflicts, are reasons that may explain a belief, but they are not the right sort of reasons to support a knowledge claim.

Truth is democratic in the sense that the truth of a statement, the validity of an argument, is independent of who believes it. Tyrants can keep evidence from us, but they cannot make a bad argument good. If something is a good reason for believing, say, that the earth rotates on its axis as it revolves around the sun, then it is a good reason for anybody. It makes a claim not just on the person who offers it but on everyone else. The way in which evidence and good reasons make claims on everybody, independently of their rank and interests, helps explain the connection between truth and consensus. When a statement is true, and known to be true, then, because there is evidence for its truth, there is likely to be a consensus over the long run.

Here is our view of knowledge so far. Knowledge is true, justified, belief, a view now known in Anglo-American philosophy as 'the standard view' of knowledge. This is more-or-less what Plato concluded in the *Theaetetus*. But we may be left saying: okay, this is what knowledge is. But how do we ever know *that* we know?

It is true that one can never have certainty in the sense of a guarantee against all future grounds for doubt. But if I do not know for sure that p is true, how can I know it? Wittgenstein remarks: ' "If I know something, then I also know that I know it, etc." amounts to: "I know that" means "I am incapable of being wrong about that". But whether I am so needs to be established objectively' (1972: 4e). To assert that p makes a claim; but so does asserting 'I *know* that p'. Claims are made by people, in particular circumstances, with only partial evidence; they are always open to refutation by evidence beyond the person's ken. (This is one of the reasons why any consensus among believers that counts toward knowledge must be a consensus over time.) When we think about it, we see that knowing that p, and knowing *that* one knows that p, are in the same boat: knowing *that* we know leads to an infinite regress. We find ourselves repeating the same request again and again, for making sure that I know that I know asks for no new checks to be done, only the same old ones. Apparently nothing will satisfy us, which suggests we do not know what we are asking for. We cannot be demanding that the belief in question be logically true, necessarily true, like the 'belief' that 'everything is what it is and not another thing'; for no empirical proposition can have that kind of certainty.

From Descartes to Wittgenstein our thinking about the nature of know-ledge, meaning, self-knowledge, and the *grounds* of knowledge has taken a radical turn. Descartes was looking for building blocks of knowledge. Unless these were indubitable propositions, knowledge could not get going. The building blocks he thought he found were mental images and beliefs, not about the external world but about one's own *beliefs*. These and only these, he thought, are indubitable. But, as we noted, the quest for infallibility makes no sense apropos empirical propositions. Furthermore, in the ordinary sense of the word, we can be *certain*. In the ordinary circumstance, as G. E. Moore argued, I can be certain that, when I hold up my two human hands, there are in front of me two material objects—namely, two human hands. Might some strange now unimagined circumstance call this into doubt? Possibly. But doubting, too, requires grounds, in the form of present circumstances that call the knowledge we believe we have into question. And what can count as a ground for doubting one empirical proposition can only be some other empirical proposition or set of propositions.

Cartesian certainty rests on an untenable theory of meaning that severs meaning from behavior, mind from world and other minds, and makes a mystery of the very thing we need to understand, intentionality. Recall Wittgenstein's remarks: 'If I wanted to doubt whether this was my hand, how could I avoid doubting whether the word "hand" had any meaning?' And 'If I don't know *that*, how do I know that my words mean what I think they mean?' And if I don't know that, I am not a speaker-thinker who can pose these questions in the first place.

'Knowledge is in the end based on acknowledgment,' Wittgenstein (1972: 49e) writes. The first definitions of 'acknowledge' given by *The Shorter Oxford English Dictionary* are '(1) to recognize or confess (a person or a thing to be something); own the claims or authority of . . . (2) Own with gratitude or as an obligation . . . (3) Register recognition of, take notice of . . . '. How different this idea of a base for knowledge is from Descartes's! The ground of knowledge is not to be found in indubitable propositions about the inner world, but in the ways we live in the world together. We acknowledge that with which we are already acquainted. 'Are we to say that the knowledge that there are physical objects comes very early or very late . . . The child, I should like to say, learns to react in such-and-such a way, and in so reacting it doesn't so far know anything. Knowing only begins at a later level' (Wittgenstein 1972: 63e–71e).

There is no *beginning* to knowledge in the form of particular pieces of knowledge; if we must search for beginnings, it is in the processes through which the child becomes a thinking creature. We come to have specifically human minds that can know themselves in a 'subjective' way only through inhabiting a peculiarly human form of life with other human beings, and only through a process in which we learn to read the world along lines of interest and need that we increasingly come to share with those we love. Though Wittgenstein does not say so, these forms of life are non-propositional: they both precede and, in part, generate the child's capacity for mental states of a propositional character.

Earlier I said that the possibility of consensus rests on there being a common reality to which one can refer. It is because there is something with which we are immediately in touch, in the midst of which we live, something that remains itself while being investigated from various perspectives—like the cat on the mat, or the shape of the earth, or which parent determines the sex of the embryo—that intersubjective agreement is possible, where 'intersubjective agreement' means just agreement among a number of subjects (persons) about something available to them all. And, unless we sever mind absolutely from behavior, nothing rules out the psychological life as open to intersubjective agreement in this sense: if, contra Descartes, mind and behavior are connected in essential, conceptual ways, then, though it is hard for you to determine what my feelings, intentions, and thoughts are, and though you can never be certain about them, nevertheless some are in principle discoverable over time in my behavior. The fact that speech and behavior require interpretation or a 'hermeneutic' approach does not by itself put them beyond the pale of science. In considering the mind an appropriate field for scientific investigation, Freud was suggesting ways in which mind is linked to behavior and embodied in it: parapraxes, telling a dream, recounting one's life, self-destructively repetitive actions, style, speech, rhythm of speech, bodily gestures, grimaces, frowns, sighs, groans, and other such peculiarly human gestures.

Recent psychoanalytic writers have said that 'reality' refers to something subjective, rather than to an external realm that exists independently of the subject; and that there is no such thing as an objective reality, beyond analyst and patient, that one can be 'objective' about. The passages insist that the only 'reality' we can investigate, know, deceive ourselves about must be within the realm of someone's potential experience. So Kant said, and on this point few philosophers would disagree. But it does not follow that reality is subjective. On the contrary, in the absence of a distinction between what I 'subjectively'—or even we, putting our 'subjectivities' together—believe to be the case (a belief that itself is as much a part of reality as the chair I am sitting on), and what *is* the case, however that is determined, the concept of reality loses its sense.

The analyst Charles Spezzano (1993: 30) writes: 'If an observation or measurement could establish a truth, that truth could never become untrue. Yet this happens all the time in science.' This is confused: the truth of the matter did not change; the evidence available to us did. We can do our best to have knowledge about a particular matter, can think we have achieved it, so claim to know that *p*, even feel quite certain of it; yet we may not know it. What *we take to be a truth* can always be called into question at another time, or under other circumstances. It is true that claims to truth must always be provisional; that a truth claim is always that, a claim, requiring support; that between the best evidence and *what is the case*, there will always be a gap; that a justified belief and a true belief are, unfortunately, not necessarily the same; that talk about 'the truth', especially 'sincere', self-righteous talk, is often a way of dignifying one's own blind spots; that the conversational move that says 'You're wrong' or 'That is not true' is often a conversation-stopper. All this is correct. But it is not the truth that changes, rather our beliefs.

Owen Renik (1998: 492) claims that we are 'not trying to discover something that was already present in the patient's mind but to construct a view of his life that *works*, i.e. that helps him feel better'; the analyst can rely only on his subjectivity, Renik says, and that is 'irreducible'. As an example of the analyst's irreducible subjectivity, Renik gives us the following clinical vignette. His patient, Ethan, has the impression that, as he was telling the story of saving a patient's life, Renik's attention has wandered. At first Renik thinks this is not true, and he explores with Ethan the possible motivations that might explain his erroneous belief. But, as a good interpreter of his analyst's experience, Ethan insists that Renik's attention wandered, and that this inattentiveness has reminded him of his father. Renik begins to reflect. He realizes that indeed his mind did wander, and that when it did he was recalling his wish that he could have saved his mother's life, and thinking about the part this wish played in his becoming a psychoanalyst.

It seems, then, that there are things that were discovered about this interaction—one of which was that Ethan was right in some of his perceptions.

The complicated sorts of communications that often take place between analyst and patient do sometimes raise questions about whether the analysand's thoughts are already in his mind, discoverable through analytic interpretation, or are rather created jointly through the analytic dialogue. Thomas Ogden writes about a particular kind of experience in which the analyst draws on his own musings, feelings, fantasies, and apparent wanderings of the mind, to understand what is going on at that moment in the mind of the other, and to communicate that understanding in the most effective way.

Both persons contribute to this sort of interchange, and it may have an effect on both their minds. Ogden (1994: ch. 6) describes a particular case in which he comes to understand that his patient is feeling mechanical, dead; and the highly personal, yet attuned thought processes that have allowed Ogden to reach this understanding also give him the felicitous imagery of machines and airless chambers that he spontaneously uses in talking to the patient. Ogden is not alone among contemporary analysts in calling attention to this sort of creative, interpersonal, experience.

But is the creativity of the process Ogden describes incompatible with there being something in the patient that it discovers? Surely not always; nor does Ogden suggest that it is. Yet one might mistake the creativity of the discovery process for the different idea that what it 'discovers' is itself created. In the case Ogden describes, the patient's sense of deadness is a fact about him which is presumably there independently of Ogden's interpretation, and which, though they would have expressed it differently to the patient, could have been found out by other persons in their own, equally idiosyncratic ways.

The route to discovering anything, at least anything interesting, is seldom a matter of impersonally following some standard procedure. Holmes discovered that Moriarty had committed the crime; Einstein, the general theory of relativity; Watson and Crick, together, the structure of DNA—through a process unique to each person, or pair. In each case it called for creativity. Yet in each case the discovery could have been made and verified by others; and they were discoveries, not creations or inventions. So the creativity involved in discovery does not by itself mean that there is no discovery involved. This is not to say that psychoanalytic interpretation is always a discovery. Nor that the difference between discovery and creation is always clear. Particularly where the psychoanalyst is trying to reconstruct early pre-verbal experiences, the lines between discovery, creation, and invention are blurred.

If there is no such thing as knowledge of how things objectively are, then there is also no such thing as knowledge of ourselves; for to say that my mind wandered makes a claim about myself that is presumably true, and for which not only I but also others observing me can give (not conclusive proof but) evidence. The process of self-discovery often takes at least two people; it may require all kinds of creative acts. But, to return to Renik. He and Ethan do not create or invent the fact that Renik's mind wandered. He acknowledges it. That he does is the reason, presumably, for Ethan's gratitude. Renik wants to jettison objectivity as a claim about how things really, objectively, are, and substitute for it objectivity as it pertains to purposes or goals. We are to ask not 'What is true, in this instance?' but 'What works in this instance?' Yet his clinical vignette makes clear that he too relies on objectivity in the first sense.

In making a plea for a pragmatist conception of truth—truth is what works—Renik gives the example of a man observing, while hiking through the hills, that the sun moves from east to west. An astronomer, on the contrary, observes that the sun does not move through the sky at all; rather it is the earth that moves, rotating daily on its axis while revolving yearly around the sun. These two observations apparently contradict each other. But in order to reconcile them, must we give up objectivity as a claim about how things are in the world, as Renik suggests, and resort instead to objectivity in the sense of goal? Is what makes the hiker's observation objective the fact that it permits him to navigate successfully, while the astronomer's observation is objective because it permits a rocket ship to be sent to Mars? No. It is rather that, in the context of certain goals, the difference between what works and what is true does not show up. One of the differences between saying 'This belief is true' and 'This belief works' is that the latter makes sense only given a specific goal, whereas truth is not limited to specific aims and goals.

The hiker and the astronomer do have different goals; but the discrepancy about what is the case is only apparent. Presumably our post-Copernican hiker knows that a careful statement of his observations would go something like this: 'Given my position, the sun appears to be moving across the sky from east to west.' And, given the hiker's position, so it does appear. It is an objective statement of fact, one that can be verified by anyone else in a similar position.

Suppose now that the hiker does not know what the astronomer knows about the universe. The hiker insists not merely that the sun appears from a certain point of view to move across the sky from east to west, but that it does in fact move that way—that is, that it would so appear from any point of view. If so, the hiker is mistaken. But let us suppose he is not so parochially intransigent; imagine him as a curious child or denizen from a pre-scientific culture. Say also that we teach him what our astronomer knows: we show him what can be seen through a powerful telescope; we construct a model of the solar system that displays how the sun looks from different positions in space; we explain to him how this model comprehends both his earlier impressions and the astronomer's. After this teaching, the child or the informant might say, 'I now see that my claim was not objective. It didn't take into account what can be seen from other points of view. My claim was made from too narrow a base.'

'But we always see things from a narrow base,' the relativist might respond. 'There is always the possibility of a more inclusive view.' This is right. But now he goes on: 'So therefore every viewpoint is as much or as little objective as every other.' Here the relativist gets careless. Let me try to bring this out by supposing the following. We have shown our pre-Copernican hiker the telescope, and our model of the solar system, and even taken him up in a rocket ship. And he says, 'Well so what! None of us knows anything for certain.' Or he insists, 'Well, since my observations work perfectly well for me, they're just as good as yours. They're right for me.' At this point what might be taken for modesty under some circumstances—'All I know is my experience'—looks more like arrogance.

I necessarily bring myself and my particular angle on the world with me wherever I go; but the relativist overlooks the fact that I can go to different places, and that when I do I may see things I did not see before. Furthermore, I can put together my new impressions with my earlier, more partial view. This is what we do when we integrate our feelings and experiences. As describing an attitude, objectivity means something like this: the awareness that perspectives other than the ones available to me up to now are relevant to determining the truth, together with an openness to discovering those perspectives for myself. The analyst's subjectivity is irreducible only in the sense that each of us perceives what he or she does from an idiosyncratic position that includes not only her location in space and time, but also her particular (partly shared) vocabulary, her conceptual repertoire, her set of skills, talents, and sensitivities, her psychological history, and so on. Every view is partial; there is no such thing as a view from everywhere, or nowhere.

Here is a clinical vignette of my own. On a particular occasion a patient was suddenly annoying me. Perhaps she was, though unconsciously, out to annoy me, perhaps to get me to scold her and punish her. But I had the sense that my feelings had little to do with her. She was their stimulus, not their content. When I described this incident to a friend, she remarked that my patient sounds a lot like my mother, about whom I had recently been complaining. My friend's remark was illuminating, and suddenly my annoyance made sense.

What allowed my friend to see something very obvious about me that I did not see? A direct line to The Truth that I lacked? Rather, the fact that she has a different point of view on me from my own, one less involved with my mother, among other things. What point of view did my friend adopt in seeing what she saw about me? My point of view? Not exactly. Did she give up her own? Not that either. Her point of view was hers, but it imaginatively embraced me and mine.

At his best, our scientifically naive hiker, I earlier suggested, is open to learning about points of view other than the one he started out with. Is not this process a little like something that happens in therapy? We try—we as both analysts and patients—to recognize how it is we see the world, to locate and understand the experiences that have convinced us that the world and we ourselves are a certain way; we ask ourselves sometimes whether we really know what we think we know, or whether we merely assume it. Later we may discover that some defensive purpose is at work in our perceptions. We begin to recognize, perhaps, the childhood perspective from which many of our perceptions are formed, a perspective that was defined by our needs, our feelings, by what we could know of the people around us at the time. The hope is that, as our need to perceive in the way we habitually do becomes less urgent, aspects of the world that were hidden from us become manifest. In this larger picture our earlier impressions will themselves look rather different. A transforming integration has taken place. The understanding at which we may arrive in these ways is more objective in that it takes more things that are relevant into account; it is formed from a point of view from which not all but more things can be considered.

Renik asks how an analyst can be objective if his view is irreducibly subjective. It is an odd question, for why should the fact that I observe an object from a particular perspective imply that I do not observe how it really is? Some things can be seen only from a particular point of view. For example: if you are unable to follow two or more musical lines, you will not be able to hear the voices in a fugue; if you do not know about protists, you may not notice the differences between a ciliate and a flagellate. Vice as well as skill can serve perception: if you are a hypocrite, a coward, or an inveterate self-deceiver, you may better be able to detect the tones of hypocrisy and self-deception, than someone of nobler character.

Gadamer (1977: 9) puts the point this way:

Prejudices are not necessarily unjustified and erroneous, so that they inevitably distort the truth. In fact, the historicity of our existence entails that prejudices, in the literal sense of the word, constitute the initial directedness of our whole ability to experience. Prejudices are biases of our openness to the world. They are simply conditions whereby we experience something—whereby what we encounter says something to us. This formulation certainly does not mean that we are enclosed within a wall of prejudices and only let through the narrow portals those things that can produce a pass saying, 'Nothing new will be said here.'

Some of the things each of us brings or fails to bring to an experience may sharpen perception; some may stunt it. So Freud spoke of repeating rather than remembering, acting out a conflict rather than recognizing it. Simple inattention and habit are also blinding: we see only what it is easy to see, what we are fully prepared to see. In their different ways, artists and psychoanalysts share the project of releasing us to perceptions that are less frozen in the past, and also often more troubling.

Truth is objective in the sense that the truth of a belief or statement is independent of my believing it true, or wanting it to be true. The belief might be true though painful to me. It might be true though I do not believe it, true though none of us believes it. By the same token, it might be false though we all believe it. It is, of course, not the relationship between earth and sun that changed after Copernicus, but the beliefs about the relationship.

How about truth as what works? But cannot a belief that works for me, even for all of us, turn out to be false? There have been times when virtually everybody assumed that the sex of a foetus was determined by the mother, and when consensus had it that women were less intelligent than men. These beliefs probably 'worked' to keep men in a position of superior power. If what works defines truth, it should be nonsensical to say: 'Now we know that neither of these beliefs is true.'

Furthermore, how are we going to assess what works? If someone says that a certain strategy is good for achieving a certain end, we want to know why she thinks so and what her evidence is. A philosophical story about how to get what we want cannot replace a story about how things objectively are, because it assumes it.

So what is truth? We might think that answering this would deliver all the particular truths there are. But the question seeks for clarification of the concept of truth, and this clarification will not tell us which particular propositions are worthy of belief. In short, we cannot give a definition of truth that will allow us to pick out just those propositions that are true. That would be magic. Nevertheless, we can say that truth is a property of sentences, beliefs, propositions, such that, if a person's belief that the earth is round is true, the world is round. Truth depends on the way things are, not on how people think they are or wish they were. What is true about a particular matter may be different not only from anybody and everybody's opinion about its truth, but also from its utility: a belief that works for me with regard to certain of my goals may turn out to be false. When pushed on this point, pragmatists often retort that considering the usefulness of a belief must refer to the longest possible run, and everything we will ever know about the way things are—a retort that collapses 'useful' back into 'true'.

If we cannot get rid of truth, then we cannot abandon the sorts of questions that a concern with truth asks, like: What evidence is there to think that a particular theory is true? Is it compatible with something else we hold true? Are you and I perhaps both deluded, or thinking wishfully? As Glen Gabbard (1997) has recently pointed out, the question of analytic 'objectivity' is not without its clinical implications. My guess is that, in their practice, most psychoanalysts honor the distinctions between justified belief and true belief, also between what works and what is the case. These distinctions call, however, for a different account of truth than the one some psychoanalysts have championed, often in the name of openness to other points of view. If we forgo the idea that analyst and patient share a common world, despite the differences in their experiences of it, we make the idea of interpretation unintelligible; for interpretation requires that there be public things, like the words we say, the things we do, the common room that patient and analyst inhabit, to give a common reference from which interpretation can get started, a ground for either agreement or disagreement. I cannot disagree with you about the time you arrived, for example, unless I know more or less what you mean by 'clock', 'time', 'today', and so on, and believe that we are talking, more or less, about the same thing. If we are not, then we are not disagreeing but talking past each other.

At the end of *War and Peace*, Pierre, who was a foolish tilting-at-windmills sort of fellow at the novel's beginning, has gone through baptisms of fire, war, and love. He has become a wise and happy man. Tolstoy (1942: 1230) writes:

There was a new feature in Pierre's relations with . . . the princess, with the doctor, and with all the people he now met, which gained for him the general good will. This was his acknowledgment of the impossibility of changing a man's convictions by words, and his recognition of the possibility of everyone thinking, feeling, and seeing things each from his own point of view. The legitimate peculiarity of each individual which used to excite and irritate Pierre now became a basis of the sympathy he felt for, and the interest he took in, other people. The difference, and sometimes complete contradiction, between men's opinions and their lives, and between one man and another, pleased him and drew from him an amused and gentle smile.

Perhaps the relativist is pleading for this sort of tolerance. But it is possible, as Tierno Bokar said, only on the recognition that there is something we share, and know we do.

References

ALTIERI, C. (2003). *The Particulars of Rapture: An Aesthetic of the Affects*. Ithaca, NY: Cornell University Press.

ANDERSON, M. C., et al. (2004). 'Neural Systems Underlying the Suppression of Unwanted Memories'. *Science*, 303 / 5655: 232–5.

ARLOW, J. A., and BRENNER, C. (1964). *Psychoanalytic Concepts and the Structural Theory*. New York: International Universities Press.

ATWOOD, G. S. R. (1992). *Contexts of Being*. Hillsdale, NJ: Analytic Press.

AUSTEN, JANE (n.d.). *Emma*. Edinburgh: Thomas Nelson & Sons.

BECHARA, A., et al. (1995). 'Double Dissociation of Conditioning and Declarative Knowledge Relative to the Amygdala and Hippocampus in Humans'. *Science*, 269: 1115–18.

BENJAMIN, J. (1995). *Like Subjects, Love Objects*. New Haven: Yale University Press.

BERLIN, I. (1998). 'From Hope and Freedom Set Free', in *Isaiah Berlin: The Proper Study of Mankind: An Anthology of Essays*, ed. H. Hausher and R. Hausher. New York: Farrar, Straus & Giroux.

BION, W. R. (1962). 'The Psycho-Analytic Study of Thinking'. *International Journal of Psychoanalysis*, 43: 306–10.

—— (1977). *Learning from Experience*, repr. in *Seven Servants*. New York: Jason Aronson.

—— (1988). 'A Theory of Thinking', in E. B. Spillius (ed.), *Melanie Klein Today*, i. *Mainly Theory*. London: Routledge.

BOLLAS, C. (1987). *The Shadow of the Object: Psychoanalysis of the Unthought Known*. New York: Columbia University Press.

BOWLBY, J. (1980). *Attachment and Loss*, iii. *Loss: Sadness and Depression*. New York: Basic Books.

BRAKEL, L. W. W., et al. (2000). 'The Primary Process and the Unconscious: Experimental Evidence Supporting Two Psychoanalytic Presuppositions'. *International Journal of Psychoanalysis*, 81 / 1: 553–71.

BRANDOM, R. B. (1994). *Making It Explicit*. Cambridge, MA: Harvard University Press.

BRITTON, R. (1989). 'The Missing Link: Parental Sexuality in the Oedipal Complex', in J. Steiner (ed.), *The Oedipus Complex Today*. London: Karnac Books.

—— (1998). *Belief and Psychic Reality. Belief and Imagination*. London: Routledge.

BROOKS, C. (1947). *The Well Wrought Urn: Studies in the Structure of Poetry.* New York: Cornwall Press.

BROUGHTON, R. E. (1993). 'Useful Aspects of Acting Out: Repetition, Enactment, Actualization'. *Journal of the American Psychoanalytic Association,* 41: 443–72.

BROWN, N. O. (1959). *Life against Death.* Middletown, CT: Wesleyan University Press.

BRUNER, J. (1983). *Child's Talk.* New York: Norton.

BUTLER, J. (1950). *Five Sermons.* New York: Library of Liberal Arts.

CAMPBELL, J. (1994). *Past, Space, and Self.* Boston: MIT Press.

CASSAM, Q. (1994) (ed.). *Self-Knowledge.* Oxford: Oxford University Press.

CAVELL, M. (1993). *The Psychoanalytic Mind: From Freud to Philosophy.* Cambridge, MA: Harvard University Press.

—— (1998). 'Triangulation, One's Own Mind, and Objectivity'. *International Journal of Psychoanalysis,* 79/ 1: 448–67.

—— (1999). 'Knowledge, Consensus, and Uncertainty'. *International Journal of Psychoanalysis,* 80/ 6: 1227–35.

CLYMAN, R. B. (1991). 'The Procedural Organization of Emotions: A Contribution from Cognitive Sciences to the Psychoanalytic Theory of Therapeutic Action'. *Journal of the American Psychoanalytic Association,* 39 (Supplement): 349–82.

CREWS, F. (1993). 'The Unknown Freud'. *New York Review of Books,* 55–67.

—— (1995). *The Memory Wars: Freud's Legacy in Dispute.* New York: New York Review.

CURLEY, E. (1998). *Behind the Geometric Method: A Reading of Spinoza's Ethics.* Princeton: Princeton University Press.

DAMASIO, A. R. (1994). *Descartes' Error: Emotion, Reason, and the Human Brain.* New York: Avon Books.

DAVIDSON, D. (1980a). 'Actions, Reasons, and Causes', in Davidson, *Essays on Action and Events.* Cambridge, MA: Harvard University Press.

—— (1980b). 'Mental Events', in Davidson, *Essays on Action and Events.* Cambridge, MA: Harvard University Press.

—— (1982). 'Paradoxes of Irrationality', in R. Wollheim and J. Hopkins (eds.), *Philosophical Essays on Freud.* Cambridge: Cambridge University Press.

—— (1989). 'The Conditions of Thought', in J. B. W. Gombocz (ed.), *The Mind of Donald Davidson.* Atlanta, GA: Editions Rodopi.

—— (1992). 'The Second Person'. *Midwest Studies in Philosophy,* 17: 255–67.

—— (2001). *Subjective, Intersubjective, Objective.* Oxford: Oxford University Press.

DAVIDSON, R. (2003). *Destructive Emotions: A Scientific Dialogue with the Dalai Lama,* narrated by Daniel Goleman. New York: Bantam Books.

DE SOUSA, R. (1987). *The Rationality of Emotion.* Cambridge, MA: MIT Press.

DEIGH, J. (2001). 'Emotions: The Legacy of James and Freud'. *International Journal of Psychoanalysis*, 82/6: 1247–56.

DENNETT, D. (1978). *Brainstorms.* Boston: Bradford Books.

—— (2003). *Freedom Evolves.* New York: Viking.

DEWEY, J. (1934). *Art as Experience.* New York: Minton, Balch & Company.

—— (1944). *Human Nature and Conduct.* New York: Henry Holt & Co.

DOSTOEVSKI, F. (1972). *Notes from Underground.* London: Penguin.

DUVALL, Y. (2005). 'Reconsolidation: State of the Union Update'. Paper delivered at NYU Cognitive Neuroscience Journal Club, 15 Apr.

EDELMAN, G. E. (1992). *Brilliant Air, Bright Fire.* New York: Basic Books.

EKMAN, P. (1998). Introduction, in *The Expression of the Emotions in Man and Animals.* Oxford: Oxford University Press.

—— and DAVIDSON, R. (1994). *The Nature of Emotions, Fundamental Questions.* New York: Oxford University Press.

ELSTER, J. (1999). *Alchemies of the Mind.* Cambridge: Cambridge University Press.

EMDE, R. (1983). 'The Representational Self', in *The Psychoanalytic Study of the Child*, vol. 38. New Haven: Yale University Press.

EPSTEIN, M. (1995). *Thoughts without a Thinker.* New York: Basic Books.

ERDELYI, M. (1974). 'A New Look at the New Look: Perceptual Defense and Vigilance'. *Psychological Review*, 81: 1–25.

EVANS, G. (1982). *The Varieties of Reference.* Oxford: Oxford University Press.

FERENCZI, S. (1956). 'Stages in the Development of the Dense of Reality', in Ferenczi, *Sex in Psychoanalysis*, trans. C. Newton. New York: Dover.

—— (1980). 'A Confusion of Tongues between Adults and the Child', in Ferenczi, *Final Contributions to the Problems and Methods of Psychoanalysis.* New York: Bruner Mazel.

FLAUBERT, G. (1965). *Madame Bovary*, trans. M. Marmur. New York: Penguin Books.

FOGEL, G. I., et al. (1996). 'A Classic Revisited: Loewald on the Therapeutic Action of Psychoanalysis. *Journal of the American Psychoanalytic Association*, 44: 863–924.

FONAGY, P. (1989). 'On Tolerating Mental States: Theory of Mind in Borderline Personality'. *Bulletin of the Anna Freud Centre.* 12: 91–115.

—— (1996a). 'Playing with Reality: I. Theory of Mind and the Normal Development of Psychic Reality'. *International Journal of Psychoanalysis*, 77: 217–33.

—— (1996b). 'Playing with Reality: II. The Development of Psychic Reality from a Theoretical Perspective', *International Journal of Psychoanalysis*, 77: 459–79.

FRANK, A. (1969).'The Unrememberable and the Unforgettable'. *Psychaoanalytic Study of the Child*, 24: 48–77.

FRANKFURT, H. (1988). *The Importance of What We Care About*. New York: Cambridge University Press.

FREUD, A. (1936). *The Ego and the Mechanisms of Defense*. New York: International Universities Press.

FREUD, S. (1893–5). *Studies on Hysteria*, repr. in The Standard Edition of the Complete Psychological Works of Sigmund Freud, 2. London: Hogarth Press.

—— (1896).'The Aetiology of Hysteria', repr. in The Standard Edition of the Complete Psychological Works of Sigmund Freud, 3. London: Hogarth Press.

—— (1897). 'Letter No. 61', repr. in The Standard Edition of the Complete Psychological Works of Sigmund Freud, 1. London: Hogarth Press.

—— (1899). *Screen Memories*, repr. in The Standard Edition of the Complete Psychological Works of Sigmund Freud, 3. London: Hogarth Press.

—— (1900). *The Interpretation of Dreams*, repr. in The Standard Edition of the Complete Psychological Works of Sigmund Freud, 5. London: Hogarth Press.

—— (1909). *Notes on a Case of Obsessional Neurosis*, repr. in The Standard Edition of the Complete Psychological Works of Sigmund Freud, 10. London: Hogarth Press.

—— (1911). 'Formulations on the Two Principles of Mental Functioning', repr. in The Standard Edition of the Complete Psychological Works of Sigmund Freud, 12. London: Hogarth Press.

—— (1914). 'Remembering, Repeating, and Working Through', repr. in The Standard Edition of the Complete Psychological Works of Sigmund Freud, 12. London: Hogarth Press.

—— (1915a).'The Unconscious', repr. in The Standard Edition of the Complete Psychological Works of Sigmund Freud, 14. London: Hogarth Press.

—— (1915b). 'Instincts and their Vicissitudes', repr. in The Standard Edition of the Complete Psychological Works of Sigmund Freud, 14. London: Hogarth Press.

—— (1916). *Introductory Lectures on Psycho-Analysis*, repr. in The Standard Edition of the Complete Psychological Works of Sigmund Freud, 15. London: Hogarth Press.

—— (1917). 'Mourning and Melancholia', repr. in The Standard Edition of the Complete Psychological Works of Sigmund Freud, 17. London: Hogarth Press.

—— (1919). 'The Uncanny', repr. in The Standard Edition of the Complete Psychological Works of Sigmund Freud, 17. London: Hogarth Press.

FREUD, S. (1920). 'Beyond the Pleasure Principle', repr. in The Standard Edition of the Complete Psychological Works of Sigmund Freud, 18. London: Hogarth Press.

—— (1923). *The Ego and the Id*, repr. in The Standard Edition of the Complete Psychological Works of Sigmund Freud, 19. London: Hogarth Press.

—— (1924). 'A Note upon the Mystic Writing-Pad', repr. in The Standard Edition of the Complete Psychological Works of Sigmund Freud, 19. London: Hogarth Press.

—— (1925). 'Negation' , repr. in The Standard Edition of the Complete Psychological Works of Sigmund Freud, 19. London: Hogarth Press.

—— (1926). 'Inhibitions, Symptoms and Anxiety', repr. in The Standard Edition of the Complete Psychological Works of Sigmund Freud, 20. London: Hogarth Press.

—— (1927). *The Future of an Illusion*, repr. in The Standard Edition of the Complete Psychological Works of Sigmund Freud, 21. London: Hogarth Press.

—— (1933). *New Introductory Lectures on Psycho-Analysis*, repr. in The Standard Edition of the Complete Psychological Works of Sigmund Freud, 22. London: Hogarth Press.

—— (1937). 'Constructions in Analysis', repr. in The Standard Edition of the Complete Psychological Works of Sigmund Freud. 23. London: Hogarth Press.

—— (1940). 'Splitting of the Ego in the Process of Defense', repr. in The Standard Edition of the Complete Psychological Works of Sigmund Freud, 23. London: Hogarth Press.

—— (1940). 'An Outline of Psycho-Analysis', repr. in The Standard Edition of the Complete Psychological Works of Sigmund Freud, 23. London: Hogarth Press.

GABBARD, G. O. (1997). 'A Reconsideration of Objectivity in the Analyst'. *International Journal of Psychoanalysis*, 78: 15–27.

GABRIELI, J. (2004). 'Research on the Relation of Psychoanalysis and Neuroscience: Function MRI Studies on the Regulation of Emotion and Memories'. The Annual Meeting of the American Psychoanalytic Association, San Francisco, CA.

GADAMER, H.-G. (1975). *Truth and Method*. New York: Crossroad Publishing Company.

—— (1977). 'The Universality of the Hermeneutical Problem', in Gadamer, *Philosophical Hermeneutics*, trans. and ed. D. E. Linge. Berkeley and Los Angeles: University of California Press.

GASSNER, S. (2001). 'The Central Role of Pathogenic Expectations and Beliefs in a Case of Intense Genital Damage Anxiety'. *Psychoanalytic Psychology*, 18/1: 92–119.

GOLDIE, P. (2000). *The Emotions: A Philosophical Exploration*. Oxford: Oxford University Press.

GOPNIK, A., and MELTZOFF, A. (1997). *Words, Thoughts, and Theories*. Cambridge, MA: MIT Press.

GORDON, R. M. (1987). *The Structure of Emotions*. New York: Cambridge University Press.

GORNICK, V. (2003). *The Situation and the Story*. New York: Farrar, Straus & Giroux.

GREEN, A. (1993). *On Private Madness*. Madison: International Universities Press.

GRICE, P. (2003). 'Meaning', in J. Baillie (ed.), *Contemporary Analytic Philosophy*. Englewood Cliffs, NJ: Prentice Hall.

GRIFFITHS, P. E. (1997). *What Emotions Really Are: The Problem of Psychological Categories*. Chicago: University of Chicago Press.

GROSSMAN, L. (1996). ' "Psychic Reality" and Psychic Testing'. *International Journal of Psychoanalysis*, 77: 508–17.

HAACK, S. (1999). 'Staying for an Answer: The Untidy Process of Groping for Truth'. *Times Literary Supplement*, 19 July, pp. 12–14.

HALL, S. (1999). 'Fear Itself'. *New York Times Magazine*, 28 Feb., pp. 227–66.

HANLY, C. (1999). 'Subjectivity and Objectivity in Psychoanalysis'. *Journal of the American Psychoanalytic Association*, 47/2: 427–45.

HEIDEGGER, M. (1962). *Being and Time*. New York: Harper & Row.

HOFFMAN, I. Z. (1983). 'The Patient as Interpreter of the Analyst's Experience'. *Contemporary Psychoanalysis*, 19: 389–422.

HOLT, R. R. (1967). 'The Development of the Primary Process: A Structural View', in R. R. Holt (ed.), *Motives and Thought: Essays in Honor of David Rapaport*. New York: International Universities Press.

HUME, D. (1951). *A Treatise of Human Nature*. Oxford: Oxford University Press.

JAMES, W. (1884). 'What Is an Emotion?' *Mind*, 9: 188–205.

—— (1961). *Psychology: The Briefer Course*. New York: Harper & Row.

JANET, P. (1919–25). *Les Meditations psychologiques*. 3 vols. Paris: Felix Alcan.

KANT, I. (1949). *The Critique of Pure Reason*, trans. F. M. Müller. New York: Macmillan.

KAPLAN-SOLMS, K., and SOLMS, M. (2000) *Clinical Studies in Neuro-Psychoanalysis*. London: Karnac Books.

KAYE, K. (1982). *The Mental and Social Life of Babies: How Parents Create Persons*. Chicago: University of Chicago Press.

KERMODE, F. (1966). *The Sense of an Ending*. Oxford, Oxford University Press.

KERNBERG, O. (1993). 'Convergences and Divergences in Contemporary Psychoanalytic Technique'. *International Journal of Psychoanalysis*, 74: 659–73.

KIHLSTROM, J. F. (1987). 'The Cognitive Unconscious'. *Science*, 237: 1445–52.

KIRKPATRICK, R. and WILLIAMS, F. (1960). 'Introduction', to J.-P. Sartre, *The Transcendence of the Ego*. New York: Hill and Wang.

KNIGHT, R. P. (1946). 'Determinism, "Freedom", and Psychotherapy'. *Psychiatry*, 9: 251–62.

KRIPKE, S. A. (1982). *Wittgenstein on Rules and Private Language*. Cambridge, MA: Harvard University Press.

LAUB, D. and AVERHAHN, N. (1993). 'Knowing and Not Knowing Massive Psychic Trauma: Forms of Traumatic Memory', *International Journal of Psychoanalysis*, 74: 287–302.

LEAR, J. (1990). *Love and its Place in Nature*. New York: Farrar, Straus, & Giroux.

——(1993). 'An Interpretation of Transference'. *International Journal of Psychoanalysis*, 74: 739–55.

LEDOUX, J. (1996). *The Emotional Brain: The Mysterious Underpinnings of Emotional Life*. New York, Simon & Schuster.

——(1998) (ed.). *The Emotional Brain*. New York: Touchstone.

——(2002) (ed.). *Synaptic Self*. New York: Viking Penguin.

LEWIS, T., AMINI, FARI, and LANNON, R. (2000). *A General Theory of Love*. New York: Vintage Books.

LOEWALD, H. (1976). 'Perspectives on Memory', in M. Gill and P. Holzman (eds.), *Psychology versus Metapsychology: Psychoanalytic Essays in Memory of George S. Klein*. New York: International Universities Press.

——(1980*a*). 'The Experience of Time', in *Hans W. Loewald: Papers on Psychoanalysis*. New Haven: Yale University Press.

——(1980*b*). 'Some Considerations on Repetition and Repetition Compulsion', in *Hans W. Loewald: Papers on Psychoanalysis*. New Haven: Yale University Press.

McGINN, C. (1999). 'Freud under Analysis'. *New York Review of Books* (Nov.).

MASSON, J. (1984). *The Assault on Truth*. New York: Farrar, Straus, & Giroux.

MEAD, G. H. (1934). *Mind, Self, and Society*. Chicago: University of Chicago Press.

MELTZER, A. N., and PRINZ, W. (2002) (eds.). *The Imitative Mind: Development, Evolution and Brain Bases*. Cambridge: Cambridge University Press.

MERLEAU-PONTY, M. (1962). *The Phenomenology of Perception*. London: Routledge & Kegan Paul.

MITCHELL, S. A. (1988). *Relational Concepts in Psychoanalysis: An Integration*. Cambridge, MA: Harvard.

MODELL, A. H. (1990). *Other Times, Other Realities*. Cambridge, MA: Harvard University Press.

MOORE, G. E. (2003). 'Proof of the Existence of the External World', in J. Baillie (ed.), *Contemporary Analytic Philosophy*. Englewood Cliffs, NJ: Prentice Hall.

MORAN, R. (1988). 'Making Up Your Mind: Self-Interpretation and Self-Constitution'. *Ratio*, NS 135–51.

—— (2001). *Authority and Estrangement*. Princeton: Princeton University Press.

NAGEL, T. (1983). 'The Objective Self', in C. Ginet and S. Shoemaker (eds.), *Knowledge and Mind: Philosophical Essays*. Oxford: Oxford University Press.

NEIMAN, SUSAN (2002). *Evil in Modern Thought*. Princeton: Princeton University Press.

NEISSER, U. (1967). *Cognitive Psychology*. Englewood Cliffs, NJ: Prentice Hall.

NIETZSCHE, F. (1956). *The Genealogy of Morals*, in Nietzsche, *The Birth of Tragedy and the Genealogy of Morals*. New York: Doubleday & Company.

—— (1974). *The Gay Science*, trans. W. Kaufmann. New York: Vintage Books.

NOZICK, R. (1981) *Philosophical Explanations*. Cambridge, MA: Harvard University Press.

NUSSBAUM, M. C. (2001). *Upheavals of Thought: The Intelligence of Emotions*. Cambridge: Cambridge University Press.

OGDEN, T. (1994). *Subjects of Analysis*. Northvale, NJ: Jason Aronson.

O'SHAUGHNESSY, E. (1988). 'Bion's Theory of Thinking and Child Analysis', in E. B. Spillius (ed.), *Melanie Klein Today*. ii. *Mainly Practice*. London: Routledge, 177–99.

PAYNE, J. D., NADEL, L., BRITTON, W. B., and JACOBS, W. J. (2002). 'The Biopsychology of Trauma and Memory', in D. Reisberg and P. Hertel (eds.), *Memory and Emotion*. New York: Oxford University Press.

PIERS, C. P. (2004). *Emergence: When a Difference in Degree Becomes a Difference in Kind.*, Stockbridge, MA: Rapaport-Klein Study Group.

PLATO (1973). *Theaetetus*. Oxford: Oxford University Press.

POLANYI, M. (1958). *Personal Knowledge*. Chicago: University of Chicago Press.

PREMACK, D., and PREMACK, A. (2003). *Original Intelligence: Unlocking the Mystery of Who We Are*. New York: McGraw-Hill.

PROUST, M. (1981). *Remembrance of Things Past*, iii. New York: Random House.

QUINE, W. V. (1961). 'Two Dogmas of Empiricism', in Quine, *From a Logical Point of View*. Cambridge, MA: Harvard University Press.

RAPAPORT, D. (1951). 'Toward a Theory of Thinking', in *Organization and Pathology of Thought*. New York: Columbia University Press.

—— (1967). 'On the Psychoanalytic Theory of Thinking', in *The Collected Papers of David Rapaport*, ed. M. M. Gill. New York: Basic Books.

REICH, W. (1949). *Character Analysis*. New York: Farrar, Straus, & Giroux.

REID, T. (1969). *Essays on the Intellectual Powers of Man.* Cambridge, MA, MIT Press.

RENIK, O. (1998). 'The Analyst's Subjectivity and the Analyst's Objectivity'. *International Journal of Psychoanalysis,* 79/3: 487–99.

RICOEUR, P. (1984). *Time and Narrative,* i. Chicago: University of Chicago Press.

——(1992). *Oneself as Another,* trans. K. Blamey. Chicago: University of Chicago Press.

RORTY, R. (1979). *Philosophy and the Mirror of Nature.* Princeton: Princeton University Press.

——(1998). 'Davidson between Wittgenstein and Tarsky'. *Critica: Revista hispanoamericana de filosofia,* 30/88: 49–71.

RYCROFT, C. (1962). *Imagination and Reality: Psychoanalytic Essays 1951–1961.* New York: International Universities Press.

SARTRE, J.-P. (1948). *The Emotions, Outline of a Theory.* New York: Philosophical Library.

——(1956). *Being and Nothingness.* New York: Philosophical Library.

——(1960). *The Transcendence of the Ego.* New York: Hill & Wang.

——(1965). *The Philosophy of Jean-Paul Sartre.* New York: Random House.

SCHACHTEL, E. G. (1959). *Metamorphosis on the Development of Affect, Attention, and Memory.* New York: Basic Books.

SCHACTER, D. (1996). *Searching for Memory.* New York: Basic Books.

SCHAFER, R. (1976). *A New Language for Psychoanalysis.* New Haven: Yale University Press.

——(1980). *Narrative Actions in Psychoanalysis.* Worcester, MA: Clark University Press.

——(1982). *The Analytic Attitude.* New York: Basic Books.

SELLARS, W. (1956). 'Empiricism and the Philosophy of Mind', in H. Feigl and M. Scriven (eds.), *The Foundations of Science and the Concepts of Psychology and Psycholanalysis.* Minnesota Studies in the Philosophy of Science, 1. Minneapolis: University of Minnesota Press.

SHAPIRO, D. (2000). *Dynamics of Character.* New York: Basic Books.

SHEVRIN, H., et al. (1996). *Conscious and Unconscious Processes: Psychodynamic, Cognitive, and Neurophysiological Convergences.* New York: Guilford Press.

SHEVRIN, S. and DYCKMAN, S. (1980). 'The Psychological Unconscious: A Necessary Assumption for All Psychological Theory'. *American Psychologist,* 35: 421–34.

SMITH, B. (2003). 'The Interiority of Mind and the Publicity of Language'. Unpublished typescript.

SOLMS, M., and TURNBULL, O. (2002). *The Brain and the Inner World: An Introduction to the Neuroscience of Subjective Experience.* New York: Other Press.

SPENCE, D. P. (1982). *Narrative Truth and Historical Truth*. New York: W.W. Norton.

SPEZZANO, C. (1993). *Affect in Psychoanalysis, A Clinical Synthesis*. Hillsdale: NJ: Analytic Press.

SPINOZA, B. (1963), *Spinoza's Ethics, and on the Correction of the Understanding*, trans. A. Boyle, intro. T. S. Gregory. New York: Dutton.

STERN, D. (1983). 'The Early Developments of Self, of Other, and of Self with Other', in S. Kaplan (ed.), *Reflections on Self Psychology*. New York: International Universities Press.

—— (1985). *The Interpersonal World of the Infant: A View from Psychoanalysis and Developmental Psychology*. New York: Basic Books.

—— (1995). *The Motherhood Constellation: A Unified View of Parent–Infant Psychiatry*. New York: Basic Books.

STOLLER, R. J. (1979). *Sexual Excitement*. New York: Simon & Schuster.

STOLOROW, R. D. (2001). 'Cartesian and Post-Cartesian Trends in Relational Psychoanalysis'. *Psychoanalytic Psychology*, 3: 468–84.

STRAWSON, P. F. (1963). *Individuals: An Essay in Descriptive Metaphysics*. New York: Anchor Books.

—— (1974). 'Freedom and Resentment', in Strawson, *Freedom and Resentment and Other Essays*. London: Methuen.

STROUD, B. (2000). *The Quest for Reality, Subjectivism and the Metaphysics of Colour*. Oxford, Oxford University Press.

TOLSTOY, L. (1942). *War and Peace*, trans. L. and A. Maude. New York: Simon & Schuster.

TOMASELLO, M. (1999). *The Cultural Origins of Human Cognition*. Cambridge, MA, Harvard University Press.

TREVARTHAN, C. (1979). 'Instinct for Human Understanding and for Cultural Cooperation: Their Development in Infancy', in M. von Cranach, K. Foppa, W. Lepenies and D. Ploog (eds.), *Human Ethology: Claims and Limits of a New Discipline*. Cambridge. Cambridge University Press.

TRILLING, L. (1972). *Sincerity and Authenticity*. Cambridge, MA: Harvard University Press.

TYSON, P. (2000). 'The Challenges of Psychoanalytic Developmental Theory'. *Journal of the American Psychoanalytic Association*, 50/1: 19–53.

VALENSTEIN, A. F. (1923). 'On Attachment to Painful Feeling'. *Psychoanalytic Study of the Child*, 28: 365–95.

VYGOTSKY, L. S. (1962). *Thought and Language*, trans. E. Hanfmann and G. Vakar. Cambridge, MA: MIT Press.

—— (1978). *Mind in Society: The Development of Higher Psychological Processes*. Cambridge, MA: Harvard University Press.

WACHTEL, P. L. (1993). *Therapeutic Communication: Principles and Effective Practice*. New York: Guilford Press.

WEISS, J. (1993). *How Psychotherapy Works.* New York: Guilford Press.

—— SAMPSON, H., et al. (1986). *The Psychoanalytic Process.* New York: Guilford Press.

WELLMAN, H. M. (1992). *The Child's Theory of Mind.* Cambridge, MA: MIT Press.

WERTSCH, J. V. (1985). *Vygotsky and the Social Formation of Mind.* Cambridge, MA: Harvard University Press.

WESTEN, D. (1997). 'Towards a Clinically and Empirically Sound Theory of Motivation'. *International Journal of Psychoanalysis,* 78/3: 521–49.

—— (1999). 'The Scientific Status of Unconscious Processes: Is Freud Really Dead?' *Journal of the American Psychoanalytic Association,* 47/4 (Fall, 1999), 1061–1107.

—— and GALBARD, G. (2002). 'Developments in Cognitive Neuroscience: I: Conflict, Compromise, and Connectionism'. *Journal of the American Psychoanalytic Association,* 50/1: 53–99.

WHITE, R. S. (2001). 'The Interpersonal and Freudian Traditions: Convergences and Divergences'. *Journal of the American Psychoanalytic Association,* 49/2: 427–54.

WIGGINS, D. (1987). *Towards a Reasonable Libertarianism: Needs, Values, Truth.* Oxford: Blackwell.

WILLIAMS, B. (1973). *Deciding to Believe: Problems of the Self.* Cambridge: Cambridge University Press.

WILSON, A., and MALATESTA, C. (1989). 'Affect and Compulsion to Repeat: Repetition Compulsion Revisited'. *Psychoanalysis and Contemporary Thought,* 12: 265–312.

WINNICOTT, D. W. (1965). *Ego Distortion in Terms of True and False Self: The Maturational Process and the Facilitating Environment.* New York: International Universities Press.

—— (1971). *Playing and Reality.* New York: Basic Books.

WITTGENSTEIN, L. (1953). *Philosophical Investigations,* ed. G. E. M. Anscombe. Oxford: Blackwell.

—— (1958). *The Blue and the Brown Books.* New York: Harper & Brothers.

—— (1972). *On Certainty,* trans. G. E. M. Anscombe. Oxford: Blackwell.

WOLF, S. (1990). *Freedom within Reason.* Oxford: Oxford University Press.

WOLLHEIM, R. (1999). *On the Emotions.* New Haven: Yale University Press.

WONG, P. (1999). 'Signal Anxiety and Unconscious Anticipation: Neuroscientific Evidence for an Unconscious Signal Function in Humans'. *Journal of the American Psychoanalytic Association,* 47/3: 818–41.

ZEMAN, A. (2002). *Consciousness: A User's Guide.* New Haven: Yale University Press.

Index